LECTIN FREE INSTANT POT COOKBOOK

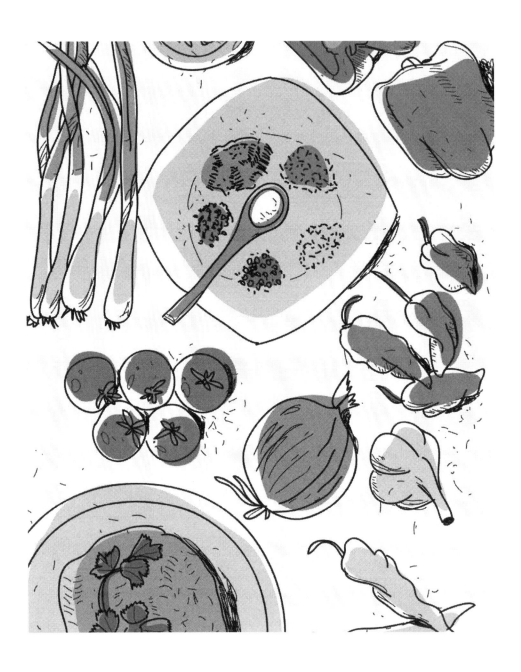

LECTIN FREE

Instant Pot

Cookbook

Top 100 Healthy and Delicious Lectin Free Recipes for Your Instant Pot

Jordan Blanc

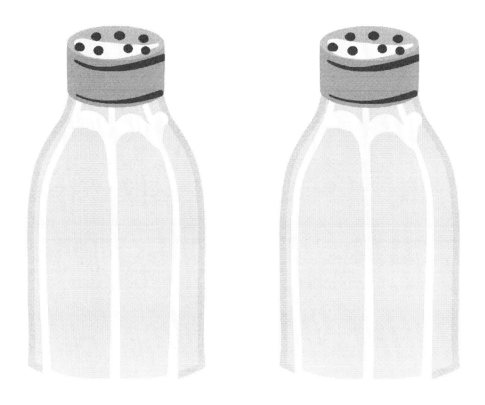

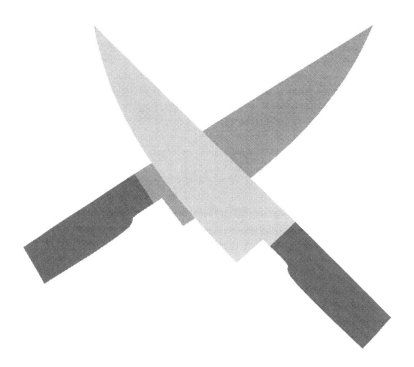

CONTENTS

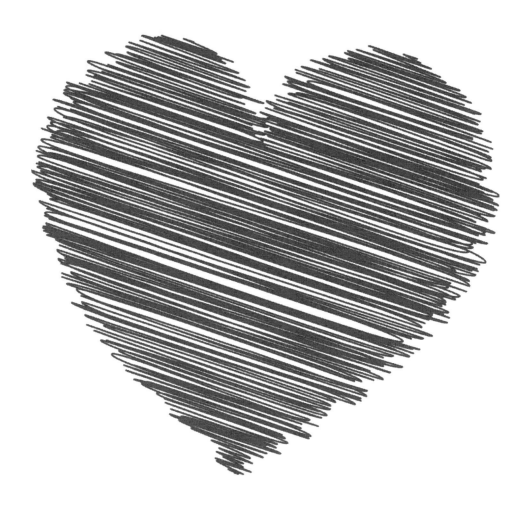

HOW I LET GO OF LECTINS

A few years ago, I noticed that I had trouble digesting certain foods, and that my digestion overall was not the same as it was before. It was making it difficult for me to enjoy food, to eat out, and even to cook on my own, because no matter what I prepared, the pain would always return and I felt sluggish after eating food.

I thought that medication would help, especially the kind that helps with digestion problems, but to no avail. Although it helped for a day or two, as soon as I started eating normally again, the pain would just return. After a while, I started carefully writing down every single thing I ate, and I also made a visit to the doctor to run some test and see what's up. As it turns out, my body has a serious issue with lectins.

I had a problem digesting many plant-based foods, such as legumes, and it was only when I removed them from my diet that everything started going back to normal. After taking it as seriously as I have, I was able to heal my digestive system, improve my overall immune system and health, and I also no longer feel any pain after eating.

However, because there are quite a few ingredients which contain lectin, cooking became a difficult thing for me to manage. I would have to balance my work life with a picky diet, which meant that I often ate nutritionally poor meals for dinner after work, even though it did not contain lectin. This is where the Instant Pot really saved me.

Once I learned how to use it properly, it was able to help me prepare delicious, lectin-free meals, and to keep them warm and fresh whenever I felt like eating. The Instant Pot was very easy to manage, and I have since become quite creative with it! I have developed my own recipes, and shared them with my friends and family, so that they too can enjoy delicious, home-made meals on the go. The thing I love most about the Instant Pot is how quickly it prepares the meals, and with how many different styles of cooking. It's amazing that so many things have been included in what looks like a simple pot. The Instant Pot has been a complete life-saver, and has made the whole process of going lectin-free much easier for me than it had ever been before.

I am now able to easily prepare any recipe with my own style of cooking, and have the cooking process both start and end whenever it suits me best. Instead of rushing home from work worrying about dinner, I now know that the Instant Pot is just waiting for me to use it! It's easy to maintain, easy to use, and so versatile in both its cooking styles and the flavors that come out of it. The Instant Pot has now become my best friend in the kitchen and I hope that you can enjoy the same benefits I have by going lectin free using your Instant Pot.

Yours in good health and happiness,

Jordan Blanc

INTRODUCTION TO THE LECTIN FREE DIET

Some of the first signs of sensitivity to lectin is problems with digestion, a painful abdomen after eating food, and also a drop in the immune system. The reason why the immune system drops is because a sensitivity to lectins means that the body does not absorb nutrients from food the way it should, meaning that people can eat, but there will not be nearly enough benefits from their food as there should be.

We will discuss every aspect of the lectin free diet in detail, both the positive and the negative sides of the diet. However, before we actually begin talking about the diet, we must first understand what lectins are, and why some people have decided to eliminate them from their diet.

WHAT ARE LECTINS?

Lectins belong to the family of proteins. More specifically, they belong to a type of protein that is derived from plants (as opposed to the protein that is found in meat). One of the main jobs of lectins is to allows cells to more easily communicate with each other. This is not their only purpose, and it is also not the only way that cells communicate, but it is the most popular way. According to some scientists, the lectins found in plants provide a form of defense by keeping insects away, which means that there are a number of uses for these proteins, as there are for others. However, some people are very sensitive to them.

For example, beans that have not been cooked properly may cause vomiting and nausea, due to a specific lectin called phytohaemagglutinin. Because the lectin has not been cooker properly, it moves itself through the digestive tracts and enters the bloodstream, causing quite the havoc.

Lectins are most often found in plants, because they contain nitrogen, which plants use to grow. The seeds of plants are the area that will have the highest amount of lectins, which is why they will especially cause problems for people who are sensitive to this protein. Lectins block the absorption of certain nutrients, causing far more work for the digestive system than it is usually used to. If untreated, the problem could lead to chronic disease, and has even been shown to cluster red blood cells together. All in all, if you are someone who is not great at handling lectins, you are far better without them. but let's look at a few more details first.

Having said that, lectins as a whole are not the bad guys. Every element in the human body has a purpose. People are sometimes sensitive to their own elements, but that doesn't mean that they will lose their intended purpose.

For example, even though lectins have so many unwanted side effects from people who cannot handle them, when it comes to lectins in small amounts, they can actually help the good bacteria, aiding digestion in the process. In controlled amounts, lectins also help the good bacteria in your gut become stronger and fight with greater force.

In some cases, research has also suggested that lectin can help to identify and diagnose cancer. Some of the most recent scientific research has actually found that lectins could potentially slow down the rate at which cancer cells multiply. This would be an incredible step for cancer research, but here it is used to show that everything in the human world has been created with an intention, even if it is not a good addition to some people's digestive system.

But for those who wish to eliminate lectin from their diet, here is more information on the topic and how lead a healthy, manageable, lectin-free life.

HOW DOES COOKING IMPACT LECTIN?

The importance of proper cooking nowhere as poignant as it is when it comes to cooking with foods that contain lectin. Cooking methods which use moist heat as the most useful when it comes to getting rid of as many lectins as possible before the food is consumed. High temperatures break down starch and simpler carbohydrates. This is great, because lectins attach themselves to carbs, and in a healthy body, would remove themselves along with the carbs as long as they can be digested. But when high moist temperatures break down the carbs, they also break down most of the lectins, which now have nothing to hold on to.

Although some people believe that cooking lentils for a long period of time will destroy the lectin protein's chain, this is not true. Lectin doesn't care how long you cook your food, as long as you cook it at very high temperatures. This is the only way to get rid of this protein and aid your digestion. It is also the reason why slow cookers are not at all recommended for those who have a problem with lectin, because pressure cooker cook food for long periods of time but at low temperatures, meaning that they do nothing to alter the chemical structure of lectin.

The best ways to drastically decrease the amount of lectins in certain foods is as follows:

- Boiling method at very high temperatures.
- Fermenting food, so that the lectins protein becomes weaker and is easily digested.
- Peeling, to remove the areas of the plant where the lectins are most likely to collect (such as the seeds).
- Pressure cooking (aka the Instant Pot), because the pressure cooker prepares food in short time intervals at very high temperatures, making it the perfect companion for a lectin-free diet.

LECTIN'S IMPACT ON YOUR HEALTH

One of the most popular supporters of the lectin-free diet is Steven Gundry, M.D., who in his books, *The Plant Paradox*, showcased that foods which contain the plant protein lectin are your worst nightmare, especially when it comes to weight loss.

The problem which needed to be overcome at a very early stage, is the fact that lectin is found in foods which people have always thought were really good for them. This includes foods such as, grains, legumes, nuts, and tomatoes. There are plenty more to join this list later on, but we just wanted to showcase the most popular ones first.

According to Gundry, the reason why humans have problems with lectins in the first place, is because humans were not intended to eat foods which contain this plant protein. Its consumption could lead to inflammation, weight gain, and an unhealthy life, specifically because the lectins drain vital nutrients which your body can no longer absorb.

FOODS YOU CAN EAT OF A LECTIN-FREE DIET

- A2 milk
- Cooked sweet potatoes
- Leafy, green vegetables
- Celery
- Garlic and onions
- Cruciferous vegetables
- Avocado
- Mushrooms
- Olives and olive oil

FOODS YOU NEED TO AVOID BECAUSE THEY ARE HIGH IN LECTIN

- Legumes
- Nightshade vegetables
- Grains
- Squash
- Fruit
- Corn
- A1 milk
- Meat from corn-fed animals

The list may seem a little bit weird until you get used to it, but it is important to follow it as clearly as possible so that the levels of lectin I your body can truly remain very low. It will never be able to completely remove lectin, because it is found in many other ingredients as well, but that doesn't mean that you cannot reduce it to the point where you can live a healthy and comfortable life.

HERE ARE THE MOST IMPORTANT HEALTH BENEFITS FROM BEING LECTIN-FREE

The main reason why scientists believe lectins should be avoided in a daily diet, is because they cause inflammations in the digestive system. The problem with this isn't that the inflammation lasts for a few hours after a lectin-heavy meal and then supposedly goes away, it's that the inflammation actually damages the walls of your intestines, making them sensitive for a long period of time. Because of this, lectins have also been known to cause autoimmune diseases such as celiac disease, diabetes, and arthritis.

But the problems don't just stop there. Gut health is strongly connected to the overall health of the rest of your body. If the food we consume somehow damages our body, it will also continue on to damage the heart, our mental health, and in the long-term, may even be the cause of cancer.

It so follows that if you were to remove lectins from your diet, you would no longer suffer from an inflamed system, which in turn would drastically reduce your risks of suffering from any of the previously mentioned illnesses. However, because lectins are present in so many other areas of our lives, we still need more research to be conducted in order to completely understand what goes on behind the mystery of lectin.

Lectins are known as sticky molecules, because they bind with sugar, causing functional shifts in the body. In small amounts, this natural shift would not be a problem. The problem arises when lectins are taken in larger quantities, especially in the kind of diet that we used to today, where everything contains highly processes grains, corn and legumes, which are generally easy to mass produce, and easy to use for the production of numerous products.

The reason why lectins cause inflammation is because they bind with the intestinal lining, especially to the villi of the small intestine. Villi, are small pockets which serve the purpose of allowing nutrients to go through them before entering the bloodstream. Essentially, villi are like little filters, which make sure that the nutrients are entering the bloodstream is the cleanest state possible, which will not interrupt the bloodstream's natural flow.

When these villi are damaged, there is nothing protecting the unfiltered nutrients from spreading throughout the body. A damaged system is highly vulnerable to bad bacteria, parasites, and pathogenic organisms. None of this is a good sign if you are trying to live a healthy life and keep your body as strong as possible.

The reason why the body eventually develops an autoimmune disease because of lectin, is because it realizes that lectins are damaging it in the long run. The way that our bodies handle harmful molecules is by creating antibodies that fight them inside our system. However, when such fights occur inside our system, the rest of the body also suffers, because every and nutrients need to be sacrificed from other areas of the body in order to win the fight. So if lectins are not removed from the diet, the process continue in a circle, causing great long-term damage to the body along the way.

A FEW DOWNSIDES TO A LECTIN-FREE DIET

Because we still need more scientific research into the world of lectins and how they affect our bodies, it is important to understand that this is certainly not everything that we must know about them.

It is not always easy to people to switch to a lectin-free diet, because there are a number of things which make that transition difficult. Namely, it is quite a restrictive diet, especially concerning foods that are use so often. This means that people will need to do a little more research into lectin-high foods, and will also need to make a detailed meal plan for the week so that they don't mistakenly eat lectins when they shouldn't be doing so.

Now, it is important to note here that excluding foods which are high in lectins doesn't mean that the entire food is bad. Every edible ingredient on our plant has at least some positive effects on our bodies, and ingredients high in lectins are no different either.

For example, grains, when eaten in moderation, can actually reduce the risks of heart disease, cancer, and diabetes. Fruits and vegetables also have many benefits for our bodies, including high vitamin and mineral levels, starch (which is important for digestion), and healthy sugars (especially at times when we are really craving something sweet). It is always better to eat whole foods than to eat anything that has been artificially produced.

A lectin-free diet will also not be easy for non-meat eaters, because so many plants are excluded from the diet, meaning that their choices of available foods are even smaller than before. This is not good, because your body needs as much of a variety of foods as possible in order to function at its optimum levels.

AND YET, THERE ARE TIMES WHEN WE SIMPLY MUST GIVE IT UP

You can reprogram your body for many things, but you cannot reprogram it for ingredients that it absolutely doesn't want anything to do with. If you were to continue to force lectins down your system, the situation would become worse and worse over time, until it reaches a point where it is no longer manageable without medication.

One of the biggest benefits of a lectin-free diet is weight loss.

A successful weight loss regime depends on a number of things, not least on making sure that your body has everything it needs to run smoothly, so that it can switch to burning excess fat. If our digestive tract is not at its optimum health levels, it cannot properly filter food, meaning that it will not focus on weight loss until it feels healthy again. If anything, your body will actually try to preserve fat so that it can use it as a source of energy later if it really must.

This is not the kind of situation you want to be in if you are trying to love weight. A lectin-free diet removes all of these problems, and leaves the body in the perfect state for weight loss and overall health developments. Many people have reported significant weight loss after switching to a diet that is very low in lectins. However, they have also noted that it takes some time for the body to first become used to the switch before any significant weight loss occurred, so it is important to remember that you must stick to it for a long period of time before you can reap any true health benefits from it. In turn, this kind of diet will also have a positive effect on your metabolism, because it will speed it up and help with even faster weight loss. But remember, you metabolism isn't just for quickly digesting food. One of its main purposes it to defend the body, make sure that it has enough heat and nutrients, and to keep it alert in various areas of life. Whether that's sports, reflect abilities, hard work, or the strength to push through heavy amounts of pressure.

THE BEST WAYS TO START A LECTIN-FREE DIET

Because we have objectively acknowledged that there are a few downsides to the lectin-free diet, which may make it a little difficult to get started, we will use this section to list as much advice and as many tips as possible, so that people can transition to a lectin-free diet without too much of a problem.

Firstly, it is important to note that whenever you are transferring diets, you should not aim to do so in a drastic manner. Suddenly dropping a huge selection of ingredients which you have been used to for years, will not result in instant health. On the contrary, it is more likely to result in cravings, bad moods, and quickly giving up before any realistic improvements have actually been made. Even lentils need not be completely eliminated from the very beginning.

The negative effects of lectin are greatly reduced through soaking and cooking the ingredients at high temperatures. This is great when it comes to ingredient such as legumes. In order to destroy the lectin inside legumes as much as possible, you can use both processes to cook them. soak the lentils in plenty of water and leave them in that water overnight. The next day, dispose of the water, add a fresh, new liquid, and begin the cooking process. Make sure that whatever liquid you are using to boil your lentils in comes up to boiling temperature for a long period of time, so that even more of the lectins can be destroyed. With this kind of cooking process, you will still be consuming lectins, but at a drastically smaller quantity, one that will probably not cause enough harm to be very noticeable.

When it comes to nightshade vegetables, such as tomatoes, eggplant, and potatoes, peeling them and de-seeding them will also do the trick of removing most of the lectins from them. lectins like to gather in the outer layer of plants, and in their seeds, more than in the actual flesh of the plant.

Similarly, when it comes to planning your food intake, you can do a lot do weigh out and prepare your food so that it contains as few lectins as possible. Many will consider this part of the process a nuisance, however, it is still something that must be done if the lectin-free diet can actually be as lectin-free as possible.

Consider planning your meals in a way where the majority of the meal will be low in lectins, even if some of it still contains a few. Your body isn't defenseless against lectin, so some of it will still be handled if it enters the system.

Make sure that you measure all of the ingredients, and that each meal still provides you with enough carbs, fat, protein, and starch, so that your body can continue to function properly. If you just eliminate foods and try to live off of those that remain, you will quickly suffer from nutritive deficiency, which is where all of the cravings and negative effects of switching to a new diet will be kicking in. Do not place yourself in this situation, because it will be incredibly difficult to get out of. Instead, focus on creating a narrowed down list of foods that you *can* have, and them make the most of those in every meal.

Another great tip is to make an imaginary meal for when you are eating out or attending a celebration. Think of the kinds of foods that you can eat in these situations, and write them down. This will make it so much easier to choose healthy options when you find yourself outside of your home, and will not cause you any embarrassment or stress in front of other people. The more you plan for your life, the easier you will find it to deal with any situation that life may place you in.

leaving things to the last second, or trying to decide on a meal order in a state of panic will cause you to choose the wrong option, and may even result in a developing a bad relationship with food.

Remember, the purpose of a lectin-free diet isn't to make you scared of food, or to completely force you to eliminate a particular ingredient. A lectin-free diet is a realistic look at what certain molecules do which is harmful to our bodies, and how to exclude those molecules as much as possible. No one expect you to be perfect on your first try with a lectin-free diet, as long as you keep learning and keep following news articles which discuss the latest research on the topic.

Another great tip is to really read the back of food labels before you make a purchase. For example, although it is obvious that a can of red beans contains red beans, it may not be so obvious that a canned soup contains a soy-based thickener. If you don't read the label in such a situation, you may think that you are eating spinach soup, when you are in fact eating both spinach and soy, which is not the right choice to make. This is the main problem with avoiding foods that are high in lectins, because they are so often used to create other ingredients, and it's not easy to run from them.

The best way to analyze any diet is to try it. If you have stomach problems, cannot lose weight, can feel that your body is going through inflammation, and even your doctor has confirmed it, then there is no reason why you shouldn't try it out. Every is different, and a lectin-free diet will work the same for you as it will for your friend, but the bottom line is that it will work. In order to make the most of the progress and to ensure that you are truly using the diet in a way which will specifically cater to your own body, the best thing to do it to write a journal of the foods you eat and how they made you feel.

INTRODUCTION TO THE INSTANT POT

The next step in a successful lectin-free diet is learning how to cook on it!

Remember how we mentioned that high-heat cooking is a great cooking method for weakening lectins? Well, there is a very handy appliance which will do just that – the Instant Pot!

The Instant Pot is a type of pressure cooker, meaning that its purpose is to cook food at high temperatures, for a much shorter period of time than the food would actually need to be cooked for in traditional ways of cooking. So for example, if a broth would usually take you 3 to 4 hours to cook properly, the pressure cooker would do the same in 45 to 90 minutes (depending on the kind of meat you used for your broth). Not only does this appliance save you time, it also ensures that your food reaches high temperatures, which destroy bacteria, unwanted toxins, and yes, lectins.

THE PERFECT COMPANION FOR A LECTIN-FREE DIET

One of the best benefits of the Instant Pot is its ability to retain delicious flavors and nutrients from whatever meals you intend to cook. This is great because it enables you to get the most out of the simplest ingredients. Instead of worrying about combining different flavors and watching the time that each ingredient takes to cook, you simply follow the instructions for the Instant Pot and you are ready to go.

What's even better is the fact that the Instant Cooker actually acts as five different kitchen appliances, all packed into a single one. It acts as a Pressure Cooker, Slow Cooker, Rice Cooker, Sauté, Steamer, and Warmer. That is a very creative number of cooking styles, all of which will ensure that the ingredients for your lectin-free diet are the best they can possibly be.

The Instant Pot comes in a few different sizes and shapes, which means that you can easily choose the one that fits your kitchen and your style of cooking the best. It takes up very little space in the kitchen, and it is also easy to store away if you will not be using it for a longer period of time.

It is not easy to juggle a busy life schedule and a cooking schedule at the same time, so it is always a pleasure when appliances such as the Instant Pot are here to help! It has a number of different settings, which control the temperature, the time of the cook, the time to start and the time to finish a meal. And because it acts as a warmer as well, you can actually set it up so that the meal is warm and ready for when you come back from work. This is such a time-saver, because all you need to do is place all of the lectin-free ingredients into the Instant Pot, and set it up to start when you are ready.

There is very little prep time for this style of cooking, and it is also a great way to save money, because you can prepare meals in larger quantities for a few days in advance. This way, you will not be rushing to grab a ready-meal when you are absolutely hungry from a long day at work, but you will instead always have something healthy prepared. You can pack your meals on the go, or separate them into containers so that they are ready for each day of the week.

Its safety features are particularly impressive, because it has been designed in such a way that it pretty much takes care of itself. For example, if for whatever reason the temperature inside the Instant Pot soared to unsafe numbers, or the pressure builds up too much, the safety mechanism inside the Instant Pot would automatically turn it off. The likelihood of this happening is incredibly small, but it is always a good feeling to know that safety has been of the utmost concern for the people who designed this appliance. It's also great for families with children, because it prevents children from getting harmed, which is a dangerous scenario for any household with boiling pots and pans.

The maintenance for this appliance is very easy. Because it is made from non-stick materials, all you need to do to clean it is to use warm water any commercial kitchen soap. There is no need for any strong chemicals, which are actually frowned upon when it comes to appliances such as the Instant Pot because they can ruin the protective layer of the pot.

The only real safety points that you as a user need to remember is to always follow the manufacturers instructions. This is true both for cleaning methods, cooking methods, and situations where something may break down. Never try to fix the Instant Pot on your own because you could ruin the delicate software and overall design of the appliance, causing it to no longer work at its optimum efficiency. Instead, always take it to a professional if you have any concerns.

But perhaps more than anything else, the Instant Pot was made not only to help families and busy people live a healthier, easier life, but to help those who are transferring to a different diet stick to it. Nothing is more frustrating than learning a whole new way of cooking and managing your food. And when stressful periods of life knock on the door, many people will instantly give up and revert back to their old ways. This is not necessarily a weakness of character, but simply an expected reaction to a very complicated way of life.

The Instant Pot keeps people interested in healthy eating because it is easy to use, comes with many tips and tricks on how to cook specific ingredients, and is also easy to clean. Every family member can enjoy their favorite meals with the Instant Pot, and they can all easily learn how to prep the food and set up the appliance so that the food is ready and warm when the first person comes home from a long day of work or school.

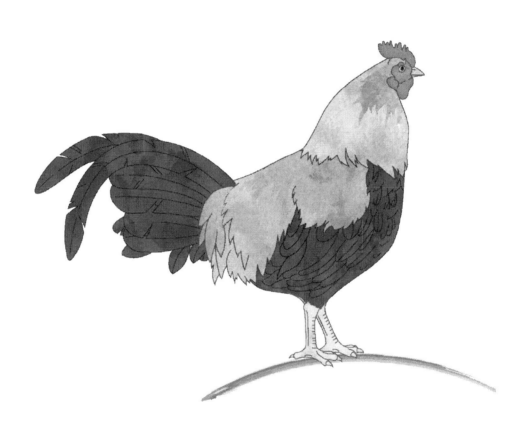

POULTRY RECIPES

Contents

Chicken Coconut Curry

Serves: 6 / Preparation time: 10 minutes / Cooking time: 15 minutes

1 ½ lbs pastured chicken thigh

1 tbsp extra virgin olive oil

1 tbsp tapioca starch

2 tbsp hot water

1 onion, diced

1 tbsp garlic, minced

1 tsp chili powder

1 ½ tbsp curry powder

1 ½ tsp dried basil

27 oz coconut milk

2 tsp sea salt

- Add oil into the instant pot and set the pot on sauté mode.
- Season chicken with salt and place in the instant pot. Sauté chicken from both sides until lightly brown.
- Remove chicken from pot and place on a plate.
- Add coconut milk, chili powder, curry powder, and basil and stir well.
- Add garlic, onion, and chicken and stir.
- Seal instant pot with lid and cook on manual high pressure for 10 minutes.
- Release pressure using the quick release method than open the lid carefully.
- Shred the chicken using a fork.
- In a small bowl, mix together tapioca and hot water and pour over chicken mixture and stir well.
- Serve and enjoy.

Per Serving: Calories: 550; Total Fat: 41.5g; Saturated Fat: 29.7g; Protein: 36.3g; Carbs: 11.8g; Fiber: 3.9g; Sugar: 5.2g

Flavourful Spiced Chicken Thighs

Serves: 6 / Preparation time: 10 minutes / Cooking time: 15 minutes

6 pastured chicken thighs

3 tbsp olive oil

¾ cup chicken stock

½ tsp garlic, minced

½ tsp ginger, minced

¼ tsp allspice

½ tsp herb de Provence

½ tsp ground coriander

½ tsp chili powder

1/8 tsp black pepper

Salt

- In a large bowl, mix together chili powder, ginger, garlic, allspice, herb de Provence, ground coriander, 2 tbsp olive oil, black pepper, 2 tbsp chicken stock, and salt.
- Add chicken in a bowl and coat well with spice mixture.
- Add remaining oil in the instant pot and set the pot on sauté mode.
- Add chicken in the pot and sauté until brown from both the sides, about 3 minutes.
- Remove chicken from pot and place on a plate.
- Add remaining chicken stock in the instant pot and stir well. Place trivet in the pot.
- Place chicken on top of the trivet.
- Seal instant pot with lid and select manual high pressure for 12 minutes.
- Allow to release pressure naturally for 10 minutes then release using the quick release method.
- Open the lid carefully and serve.

Per Serving: Calories: 340; Total Fat: 18g; Saturated Fat: 4g; Protein: 42.4g; Carbs: 0.5g; Fiber: 0.1g; Sugar: 0.1g

Lemon Garlic Chicken

Serves: 4 / Preparation time: 10 minutes / Cooking time: 15 minutes

6 pastured chicken thighs, skinless and boneless

1/3 cup chicken stock

1 lemon zest

1 lemon juice

1 ½ tbsp Italian seasoning

3 garlic cloves, minced

½ onion, chopped

3 tbsp olive oil

½ tsp chili powder

½ tsp garlic powder

Pepper

Salt

- Season chicken with chili powder, garlic powder, pepper, and salt.
- Add 2 tablespoon of olive oil in the instant pot and set the pot on sauté mode.
- Place chicken into the instant pot and sauté until brown from both the sides, about 3 minutes.
- Remove chicken from pot and place on a plate.
- Add remaining olive oil into the instant pot. Add garlic and onion and sauté for 3-4 minutes.
- Add lemon juice and cook for a minute.
- Add chicken stock, lemon zest, and Italian seasoning. Stir well.
- Return chicken into the instant pot.
- Seal pot with lid and cook on manual high pressure for 7 minutes.
- Allow to release pressure naturally for 5 minutes then release using the quick release method.
- Serve and enjoy.

Per Serving: Calories: 541; Total Fat: 28.6g; Saturated Fat: 6.3g; Protein: 64.1g; Carbs: 4.7g; Fiber: 1g; Sugar: 1.8g

Delicious Tandoori Chicken

Serves: 4 / Preparation time: 10 minutes / Cooking time: 10 minutes

1 ½ lbs pastured chicken breasts, cut into chunks

14 oz coconut milk

1 tbsp ginger, minced

½ tsp chili powder

1 tsp turmeric

1 tsp garlic powder

1 tbsp cumin

1 tbsp curry powder

½ tsp salt

- Add all ingredients into the instant pot and stir well.
- Seal pot with lid and cook on manual high pressure for 10 minutes.
- Allow to release pressure naturally for 10 minutes then release using the quick release method.
- Stir well and serve.

Per Serving: Calories: 572; Total Fat: 37g; Saturated Fat: 24.6g; Protein: 52.3g; Carbs: 9.1g; Fiber: 3.3g; Sugar: 3.6g

Perfect Shredded Chicken

Serves: 6 / Preparation time: 10 minutes / Cooking time: 12 minutes

2 lbs pastured chicken breasts

½ cup chicken stock

3 tbsp ranch dressing mix

½ tbsp ground cumin

½ tbsp chili powder

½ tbsp garlic, minced

2/3 cup Italian dressing

- Place chicken into the instant pot.
- In a small bowl, mix together Italian dressing, stock, ranch dressing mix, cumin, chili powder, and garlic and pour over chicken.
- Seal pot with lid and select manual high pressure for 12 minutes.
- Allow to release pressure naturally for 10 minutes then release using the quick release method.
- Remove chicken from pot and shred using the fork.
- Serve and enjoy.

Per Serving: Calories: 371; Total Fat: 18.9g; Saturated Fat: 4.3g; Protein: 44.2g; Carbs: 4g; Fiber: 0.3g; Sugar: 2.5g

Lemon Dill Chicken

Serves: 3 / Preparation time: 10 minutes / Cooking time: 8 minutes

6 pastured chicken thighs

2 green onions, chopped

½ cup white wine

1 tsp fresh dill weed, chopped

1 tbsp fresh lemon juice

1 lemon, sliced

¼ cup olive oil

¼ tsp black pepper

½ tsp salt

- Place chicken into the instant pot.
- Add olive oil and lemon slice on top of chicken.
- Sprinkle chicken with dill weed, pepper, and salt.
- In a small bowl, mix together white wine and lemon juice and pour over chicken.
- Seal pot with lid and cook on manual high pressure for 8 minutes.
- Allow to release pressure naturally for 10 minutes then release using the quick release method.
- Garnish chicken with green onion and serve.

Per Serving: Calories: 743; Total Fat: 38.6g; Saturated Fat: 8.4g; Protein: 85g; Carbs: 4g; Fiber: 0.9g; Sugar: 1.1g

Olive Lemon Chicken

Serves: 4 / Preparation time: 10 minutes / Cooking time: 32 minutes

8 pastured chicken thighs, bone-in, and skin-on

2 tbsp fresh parsley, chopped

5 fresh thyme sprigs

1 cup green olives, pitted

1 lemon, sliced

1 onion, sliced

3 garlic cloves, sliced

1 tbsp extra virgin olive oil

½ tsp black pepper

¾ tsp kosher salt

- Add oil into the instant pot and set the pot on sauté mode.
- Season chicken with pepper and salt.
- Add half chicken into the instant pot and cook until chicken is golden brown, about 10 minutes. Transfer chicken on a plate and repeat same with remaining chicken.
- Add garlic into the instant pot and sauté for 30 seconds.
- Add thyme, olives, lemon, and onion and cook for 2 minutes.
- Place chicken on top.
- Seal pot with lid and cook on manual high pressure for 10 minutes.
- Release pressure using the quick release method than open the lid.
- Garnish with parsley and serve.

Per Serving: Calories: 643; Total Fat: 28.8g; Saturated Fat: 7g; Protein: 85.5g; Carbs: 7.1g; Fiber: 2.3g; Sugar: 1.6g

Chicken & Mushroom

Serves: 6 / Preparation time: 10 minutes / Cooking time: 30 minutes

2 lbs pastured chicken thighs, skinless and boneless

2 tbsp red wine vinegar

½ tsp ground nutmeg

1 tsp garlic powder

2 rosemary sprigs

½ cup coconut cream

2 cups mushrooms, sliced

1 bay leaf

2 garlic cloves, minced

1 onion, diced

2 tbsp olive oil

1/2 tsp ground black pepper

1 tsp salt

- Add oil into the instant pot and set the pot on sauté mode.
- Add garlic, onion, and bay leaf and sauté for 5-8 minutes or until tender.
- Add rosemary and mushrooms and sauté for 5 minutes.
- Add chicken and seasoning and sauté until chicken is browned.
- Add vinegar and stir well.
- Add ¼ cup coconut cream and stir well.
- Seal pot with lid and cook on manual high pressure for 10 minutes.
- Release pressure using the quick release method than open the lid.
- Set pot on sauté mode until liquid comes to a simmer.
- Shred chicken using a fork. Once the liquid reduces by half then stir in remaining coconut cream.
- Serve and enjoy.

Per Serving: Calories: 391; Total Fat: 20.8g; Saturated Fat: 8g; Protein: 45.3g; Carbs: 4.5g; Fiber: 1.2g; Sugar: 2g

Flavorful Chicken Carnitas

Serves: 6 / Preparation time: 10 minutes / Cooking time: 15 minutes

2 lbs pastured chicken thighs, skinless and boneless

1 tbsp olive oil

½ cup of water

1 orange juice

3 garlic cloves, minced

1 onion, sliced

1 bay leaf

1 tsp ground cumin

½ tsp dried thyme

2 tsp dried oregano

½ tsp black pepper

1 tsp sea salt

- Add all ingredients except olive oil into the instant pot and stir well.
- Seal pot with lid and cook on manual high pressure for 10 minutes.
- Allow to release pressure naturally for 15 minutes then release using the quick release method.
- Remove chicken from pot and shred using a fork.
- Heat oil in a pan over medium heat.
- Add shredded chicken to the pan and cook until crispy, about 5 minutes.
- Serve and enjoy.

Per Serving: Calories: 327; Total Fat: 13.7g; Saturated Fat: 3.4g; Protein: 44.3g; Carbs: 4.3g; Fiber: 0.8g; Sugar: 2g

Lemon Garlic Chicken Legs

Serves: 4 / Preparation time: 10 minutes / Cooking time: 25 minutes

2 lbs pastured chicken legs

1 cup of water

6 garlic cloves, peeled

1 lemon, quartered

1 tsp Italian herb seasoning

¼ tsp black pepper

1 tsp salt

- Add water and garlic cloves to the instant pot.
- Add chicken legs into the instant pot.
- Sprinkle chicken with Italian herb seasoning, pepper, and salt. Add lemon on top of chicken.
- Seal pot with lid and cook on manual mode for 25 minutes.
- Release pressure using the quick release method than open the lid.
- Serve and enjoy.

Per Serving: Calories: 442; Total Fat: 16.9g; Saturated Fat: 4.6g; Protein: 66.1g; Carbs: 2.9g; Fiber: 0.5g; Sugar: 0.4g

Spicy Tandoori Chicken

Serves: 4 / Preparation time: 10 minutes / Cooking time: 15 minutes

2 lbs pastured chicken drumsticks	1 tbsp chili powder
1 tbsp olive oil	½ tbsp garlic, minced
1 tbsp fresh lemon juice	½ tbsp ginger, grated
1 tsp garam masala	½ cup of coconut yogurt
½ tsp turmeric	2 tsp salt

- In a large mixing bowl, add coconut yogurt, oil, lemon juice, garam masala, turmeric, chili powder, garlic, ginger, and salt and mix well.
- Add chicken in a mixing bowl and coat well with marinade and place in refrigerator for overnight.
- Pour 1 cup of water into the instant pot then place a trivet in the pot.
- Arrange marinated chicken drumsticks on a trivet.
- Seal pot with lid and cook on manual high pressure for 15 minutes.
- Allow to release pressure naturally then open the lid.
- Serve and enjoy.

Per Serving: Calories: 439; Total Fat: 17.4g; Saturated Fat: 4.3g; Protein: 63.3g; Carbs: 3.8g; Fiber: 0.8g; Sugar: 1.9g

Tasty Mediterranean Chicken

Serves: 4 / Preparation time: 10 minutes / Cooking time: 35 minutes

1 ½ lbs pastured chicken thighs	½ tsp oregano
1 onion, sliced	½ tsp mint, crushed
3 garlic cloves, minced	½ tsp onion powder
2 tbsp olive oil	1 tsp garlic powder
1 lemon juice	½ tsp black pepper
¾ cup chicken stock	½ tsp salt

- Add oil into the instant pot and set the pot on sauté mode.
- Coat chicken with all dry spices and place into the instant pot and cook until chicken is brown from both the sides, about 4 minutes a side.
- Once the chicken is browned then remove from pot and place on a plate.
- Add garlic to the pot and sauté for 30 seconds.
- Return chicken to the pot along with chicken stock and lemon juice and stir well.
- Add sliced onion on top of chicken.
- Seal pot with lid and cook on high pressure for 10 minutes.
- Release pressure using the quick release method than open the lid.
- Remove chicken from pot and place on a baking tray and broil chicken for 3 minutes per side.
- Set instant pot on sauté mode until sauce reduces, about 5-10 minutes.
- Cover chicken with sauce and serve.

Per Serving: Calories: 407; Total Fat: 19.9g; Saturated Fat: 4.6g; Protein: 50.1g; Carbs: 4.8g; Fiber: 1g; Sugar: 1.9g

Chicken Sweet Potato Curry

Serves: 4 / Preparation time: 10 minutes / Cooking time: 25 minutes

8 pastured chicken thighs

1 tsp turmeric

1 red chili, chopped

1 tsp ground ginger

1 small sweet potato

2 garlic cloves, chopped

2 carrots, chopped

7 oz chicken stock

7 oz coconut milk

2 tsp coriander, chopped

2 tsp cumin

1 onion, chopped

1 tbsp olive oil

- Using sharp knife pierce sweet potato and microwave for 5 minutes. Remove from microwave and set aside to cool.
- Add oil into the instant pot and set the pot on sauté mode.
- Add onion, ginger, carrot, and garlic into the pot and cook until softened.
- Cut sweet potato in half and scoop out all flesh.
- Add sweet potato flesh into the pot along with spices. Mix well.
- Add chicken thighs, chicken stock, coconut milk, and chili and stir well.
- Seal pot with lid and cook on manual high pressure for 15 minutes.
- Allow to release pressure naturally then open the lid.
- Shred the chicken using a fork and stir well into the sauce.
- Garnish with chopped coriander and serve.

Per Serving: Calories: 748; Total Fat: 37.5g; Saturated Fat: 17g; Protein: 87g; Carbs: 13.2g; Fiber: 3.3g; Sugar: 5.5g

Juicy Turkey Breast

Serves: 10 / Preparation time: 10 minutes / Cooking time: 30 minutes

6 lbs pastured turkey breast

1 onion, peeled and quartered

1 celery rib, cut into 1-inch pieces

1 tsp thyme

1 1/2 cups chicken stock

Pepper

Salt

- Pour stock into the instant pot.
- Add celery, onion, and thyme into the pot.
- Season turkey breast with pepper and salt.
- Place trivet into the instant pot then place turkey breast on a trivet.
- Seal pot with lid and cook on manual high pressure for 30 minutes.
- Allow to release pressure naturally then open the lid.
- Transfer turkey breast on a serving dish.
- Slices and serve.

Per Serving: Calories: 290; Total Fat: 4.6g; Saturated Fat: 0.9g; Protein: 46.7g; Carbs: 12.8g; Fiber: 1.7g; Sugar: 10.2g

Delicious Chicken Shawarma

Serves: 6/ Preparation time: 10 minutes / Cooking time: 15 minutes

1 1/2 lbs pastured chicken breasts, skinless and boneless

1/2 lb pastured chicken thighs, skinless and boneless

1 tsp allspice

1/4 tsp garlic, minced

1/2 tsp turmeric

1 cup chicken stock

1/8 tsp ground cinnamon

1/2 tsp chili powder

1 tsp black pepper

- Cut chicken thighs and chicken breast into strips and place in instant pot.
- In a small bowl, combine together all spices.
- Sprinkle spice mixture over the chicken. Mix well.
- Pour stock over chicken.
- Seal pot with lid and cook on poultry mode for 15 minutes.
- Allow to release pressure naturally then open the lid.
- Serve with veggies and enjoy.

Per Serving: Calories: 231; Total Fat: 9.2g; Saturated Fat: 2.4g; Protein: 34.6g; Carbs: 0.9g; Fiber: 0.3g; Sugar: 0.2g

Herb Chicken

Serves: 4 / Preparation time: 10 minutes / Cooking time: 10 minutes

1 1/2 lbs pastured chicken breasts, skinless and boneless

2 garlic clove, minced

1 tbsp olive oil

1 tsp dried basil

4 oz capers, drained

3/4 cup chicken stock

1 tsp dried oregano

1/4 cup lemon juice

Pepper

Salt

- Add olive oil into the instant pot and set the pot on sauté mode.
- Season chicken with pepper and salt.
- Place chicken into the pot and sauté until lightly brown on all sides.
- Remove chicken from pot and place on a plate.
- Add garlic and sauté for a minute.
- Add stock, basil, oregano, and lemon juice and stir well.
- Return chicken into the pot and top with capers.
- Seal pot with lid and cook on high pressure for 10 minutes.
- Release pressure using quick release method than open the lid.
- Serve and enjoy.

Per Serving: Calories: 369; Total Fat: 16.6g; Saturated Fat: 4.2g; Protein: 50.3g; Carbs: 2.6g; Fiber: 1.2g; Sugar: 0.6g

Tangerine Lemon Chicken

Serves: 2 / Preparation time: 10 minutes / Cooking time: 15 minutes

1 lb pastured chicken thighs

2 tbsp lemon juice

1/8 tsp thyme, dried

1/2 cup tangerine juice

1 tsp garlic, minced

1/2 tsp fresh rosemary, chopped

2 tbsp white wine

Pepper

Salt

- Place chicken into the instant pot.
- In a bowl, mix together tangerine juice, garlic, white wine, lemon juice, thyme, rosemary, pepper, and salt.
- Pour bowl mixture over the chicken.
- Seal pot with lid and cook on high pressure for 15 minutes.
- Allow to release pressure naturally. Open lid carefully.
- Serve and enjoy.

Per Serving: Calories: 473; Total Fat: 17g; Saturated Fat: 4.8g; Protein: 66.3g; Carbs: 7.4g; Fiber: 0.7g; Sugar: 6g

Flavorful Herb Chicken Wings

Serves: 4 / Preparation time: 10 minutes / Cooking time: 10 minutes

2 lbs pastured chicken wings

3 tbsp olive oil

1 tbsp basil

1 tbsp oregano

3 tbsp tarragon

1 tbsp chicken seasoning

6 tbsp chicken stock

1 tbsp garlic paste

Pepper

Salt

- Add all ingredients into the large bowl and mix well.
- Pour 1 cup water into the instant pot then place a trivet in the pot.
- Place marinated chicken on top of the trivet.
- Seal pot with lid and cook on high pressure for 10 minutes.
- Release pressure using the quick release method than open the lid carefully.
- Serve and enjoy.

Per Serving: Calories: 533; Total Fat: 27.6g; Saturated Fat: 6.2g; Protein: 66.3g; Carbs: 2.2g; Fiber: 0.6g; Sugar: 0.1g

Chili Orange Turkey Legs

Serves: 4 / Preparation time: 10 minutes / Cooking time: 25 minutes

2 pastured turkey legs

1/2 tsp black pepper

2 tbsp orange zest

2 tbsp chili sauce

1/2 cup orange juice

1 cup chicken stock

1 green chili, chopped

2 green onions, chopped

1 tsp sea salt

- Season turkey legs with pepper and salt and place into the instant pot.
- Pour stock over turkey legs.
- Seal pot with lid and cook on high for 15 minutes.
- Release pressure using quick release method than open the lid. Set pot on sauté mode.
- Add chili sauce and orange juice. Stir well.
- Add onion, orange zest, and green chili. Stir well and cook for 10 minutes,
- Serve and enjoy.

Per Serving: Calories: 611; Total Fat: 27.7g; Saturated Fat: 8.4g; Protein: 80.4g; Carbs: 5g; Fiber: 0.7g; Sugar: 3g

Turkey Roast

Serves: 4 / Preparation time: 10 minutes / Cooking time: 55 minutes

2 lbs pastured turkey breast, skinless and boneless

1/4 cup olive oil

1 tsp black pepper

4 cups chicken stock

3 tbsp Dijon mustard

2 tsp sea salt

- Place turkey breast into the instant pot then pour chicken stock over turkey breast.
- Seal pot with lid and cook on high for 25 minutes.
- Release pressure using quick release method than open the lid.
- Remove turkey breast from the pot and set aside.
- Preheat the oven to 220 C/ 425 F.
- In a small bowl, mix together Dijon, pepper, olive oil, and salt.
- Brush turkey breast with Dijon mixture and place on a baking tray.
- Roast meat in the preheated oven for 15 minutes on each side.
- Serve and enjoy.

Per Serving: Calories: 322; Total Fat: 13.2g; Saturated Fat: 0.6g; Protein: 36.8g; Carbs: 14.2g; Fiber: 5.3g; Sugar: 7.1g

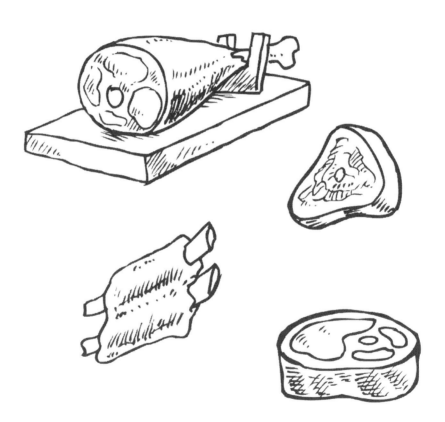

BEEF & PORK RECIPES

Contents

Beef Roast

Serves: 8 / Preparation time: 10 minutes / Cooking time: 68 minutes

3 lbs grass-fed beef chuck roast, cut into chunks

¼ cup lime juice

12 oz chicken stock

¼ cup cilantro

3 garlic cloves, minced

1 onion, sliced

2 tbsp olive oil

¾ tsp black pepper

1 tsp ground cumin

1 ½ tsp oregano, crushed

3 tbsp ancho chili powder

¾ tsp salt

- In a small bowl, mix together chili powder, cumin, oregano, pepper, and salt.
- Sprinkle spice mixture over chuck roast.
- Add oil into the instant pot and set the pot on sauté mode.
- Add meat in the pot and sauté for 6-8 minutes.
- Add garlic, cilantro, onion, lime juice, and stock and stir well.
- Seal pot with lid and cook on manual high pressure for 60 minutes.
- Allow to release pressure naturally then open the lid.
- Shred the meat using a fork and serve.

Per Serving: Calories: 660; Total Fat: 51.1g; Saturated Fat: 19.4g; Protein: 45g; Carbs: 2.7g; Fiber: 0.6g; Sugar: 0.8g

Classic Pork Carnitas

Serves: 8 / Preparation time: 10 minutes / Cooking time: 30 minutes

2 ¼ lbs pastured pork shoulder roast, cut into chunks

1 bay leaf

¼ cup fresh lime juice

1 cup of orange juice

½ tsp black pepper

1 tsp ground cumin

2 tbsp olive oil

1 tsp salt

- Add oil into the instant pot and set the pot on sauté mode.
- Season meat with pepper and salt. Place meat into the instant pot and sauté until brown.
- Add cumin, bay leaf, lime juice, orange juice, and salt and stir well.
- Seal pot with lid and cook on manual high pressure for 25 minutes.
- Allow to release naturally then open the lid.
- Remove bay leaf from pot.
- Shred the meat using a fork and stir well.
- Serve and enjoy.

Per Serving: Calories: 373; Total Fat: 29.6g; Saturated Fat: 9.5g; Protein: 21.7g; Carbs: 3.5g; Fiber: 0.1g; Sugar: 2.6g

Spicy Pork Roast

Serves: 4 / Preparation time: 10 minutes / Cooking time: 45 minutes

2 lbs pastured pork roast

1 ½ cups chicken stock

1 tsp garlic powder

½ tsp onion powder

1 tsp ground ginger

1 tbsp olive oil

1 tsp chili powder

1 tsp oregano

1 tsp thyme

1 tsp cumin

½ tsp black pepper

- Add oil into the instant pot and set the pot on sauté mode.
- In a small bowl, mix together all spices and herbs. Rub pork with spice mixture and place into the instant pot and cook until browned.
- Pour chicken stock over pork.
- Seal pot with lid and cook on high pressure for 45 minutes.
- Allow to release pressure naturally then open the lid.
- Serve and enjoy.

Per Serving: Calories: 515; Total Fat: 25.4g; Saturated Fat: 8.4g; Protein: 65.4g; Carbs: 2.5g; Fiber: 0.8g; Sugar: 0.7g

Beef Short Ribs

Serves: 4 / Preparation time: 10 minutes / Cooking time: 35 minutes

2 lbs grass-fed beef short ribs

3 tsp garlic, minced

1 tbsp ginger, grated

1/3 cup coconut aminos

1 tsp allspice

½ cup chicken broth

- Place beef ribs into the instant pot.
- Whisk together chicken broth, ginger, allspice, garlic, and coconut aminos and pour over ribs.
- Seal pot with lid and cook on high pressure for 35 minutes.
- Allow to release pressure naturally then open the lid.
- Serve and enjoy.

Per Serving: Calories: 499; Total Fat: 20.7g; Saturated Fat: 7.9g; Protein: 66.4g; Carbs: 6.1g; Fiber: 0.3g; Sugar: 0.2g

Delicious Pork Carnitas

Serves: 4 / Preparation time: 10 minutes / Cooking time: 30 minutes

2 lbs pastured pork shoulder

1 tbsp olive oil

2 tsp garlic, minced

1 tsp cumin

1 tsp oregano

2 lime juice

½ cup of water

2 cups chicken broth

1 onion, chopped

- Add oil into the instant pot and set the pot on sauté mode.
- Add meat to the pot and sauté until browned.
- Add remaining ingredients to the pot and stir well to combine.
- Seal pot with lid and cook on manual high pressure for 30 minutes.
- Allow to release pressure naturally then open the lid.
- Shred the meat using a fork.
- Serve and enjoy.

Per Serving: Calories: 733; Total Fat: 52.9g; Saturated Fat: 18.5g; Protein: 55.8g; Carbs: 5.8g; Fiber: 0.9g; Sugar: 1.9g

Tender Pulled Pork

Serves: 16 / Preparation time: 10 minutes / Cooking time: 120 minutes

6 lbs pastured pork shoulder

2 tbsp granulated garlic

2 tbsp onion powder

2 tbsp chili powder

2 tbsp cumin

1 cup chicken broth

1 tsp black pepper

1 tbsp salt

- Place meat into the instant pot.
- Add broth and spices on top of meat.
- Seal pot with lid and cook on high pressure for 2 hours.
- Release pressure using the quick release method than open the lid.
- Shred the meat using a fork.
- Season with pepper and salt and serve.

Per Serving: Calories: 512; Total Fat: 36.8g; Saturated Fat: 13.4g; Protein: 40.4g; Carbs: 2.4g; Fiber: 0.6g; Sugar: 0.7g

Tender Steak Bites

Serves: 6 / Preparation time: 10 minutes / Cooking time: 20 minutes

3 lbs grass-fed round steak, cut into bites

1 cup chicken broth

¼ cup olive oil

2 tsp garlic, minced

½ onion, diced

1 tsp black pepper

1 tsp salt

- Add all ingredients into the instant pot and stir well.
- Seal pot with lid and cook on high pressure for 20 minutes.
- Release pressure using the quick release method than open the lid.
- Serve and enjoy.

Per Serving: Calories: 574; Total Fat: 30.5g; Saturated Fat: 9.5g; Protein: 69.4g; Carbs: 1.6g; Fiber: 0.3g; Sugar: 0.5g

Healthy Beef & Broccoli

Serves: 6 / Preparation time: 10 minutes / Cooking time: 25 minutes

1 ¾ lbs grass-fed beef chuck roast, boneless and cut into chunks

1 ¼ tsp xanthan gum

12 oz broccoli florets

2 tbsp garlic, minced

2 tbsp olive oil

1 tsp ground ginger

¼ cup monk fruit sweetener

½ cup coconut aminos

1 cup chicken broth

- In a large mixing bowl, add broth, coconut aminos, sweetener, and ginger and whisk well. Add meat chunks and coat well and set aside.
- Add oil into the instant pot and set the pot on sauté mode.
- Add garlic to the pot and sauté for a minute.
- Add meat and sauce to the pot and stir well.
- Seal pot with lid and cook on manual high pressure for 15 minutes.
- Meanwhile, steam broccoli in steamer for 8-10 minutes or until tender.
- Release instant pot pressure using the quick release method than open the lid.
- Take out ¾ cup of sauce from instant pot and place in mixing bowl. Add xanthan gum to the sauce and stir until thickens.
- Return thickens sauce to the instant pot. Add steamed broccoli to the pot and stir well.
- Serve and enjoy.

Per Serving: Calories: 574; Total Fat: 41.9g; Saturated Fat: 15.4g; Protein: 37.2g; Carbs: 9.7g; Fiber: 2.3g; Sugar: 1.1g

Quick Pork Chops

Serves: 2 / Preparation time: 5 minutes / Cooking time: 14 minutes

2 pork chops

1 tbsp liquid smoke

1 cup chicken broth

1 tsp black pepper

2 tbsp olive oil

2 tsp salt

- Season pork chops from both the side with pepper and salt.
- Add oil into the instant pot and set the pot on sauté mode.
- Add pork chops to the pot and sauté until brown from both the sides, about 2 minutes each side.
- Remove pork chops from the pot.
- Add liquid smoke and broth to the pot and stir well.
- Place pork chops to the pot.
- Seal pot with lid and cook on manual high pressure for 10 minutes.
- Allow to release pressure naturally for 10 minutes then release using the quick release method.
- Serve and enjoy.

Per Serving: Calories: 398; Total Fat: 34.6g; Saturated Fat: 9.7g; Protein: 20.5g; Carbs: 1.1g; Fiber: 0.3g; Sugar: 0.4g

Kalua Pork

Serves: 8 / Preparation time: 10 minutes / Cooking time: 1 hour 30 minutes

5 lbs pastured pork roast, boneless

1 cup of water

1 onion, sliced

10 garlic cloves, peeled

1 tbsp olive oil

Pepper

Salt

- Add oil into the instant pot and set the pot on sauté mode.
- Season meat with pepper and salt.
- Place meat into the pot and sauté until brown on all sides.
- Using sharp knife make slits on roast and tuck in garlic cloves.
- Add water and onion on top of meat.
- Seal pot with lid and cook on manual high pressure for 90 minutes.
- Release pressure using the quick release method than open the lid.
- Shred the meat using fork and serve.

Per Serving: Calories: 613; Total Fat: 28.5g; Saturated Fat: 10g; Protein: 81.2g; Carbs: 2.5g; Fiber: 0.4g; Sugar: 0.6g

Coconut Pork Curry

Serves: 8 / Preparation time: 10 minutes / Cooking time: 37 minutes

4 lbs pastured pork shoulder, boneless and cut into chunks

3 cups chicken broth

2 cups of coconut milk

1 tsp turmeric

1 tbsp ground cumin

1 tbsp curry paste

3 tbsp fresh ginger, grated

3 garlic cloves, minced

1 onion, chopped

2 tbsp olive oil

Pepper

Salt

- Heat oil in a large pan over medium heat.
- Season pork with pepper and salt.
- Add meat to the pan and brown over high heat for 6-7 minutes. Transfer meat to the instant pot.
- Add onion, turmeric, cumin, curry paste, ginger, pepper, and garlic to the pan and stir well. Transfer onion mixture to the instant pot.
- Add broth and coconut milk to the pot and stir well.
- Seal pot with lid and select soup and stew mode and set timer for 30 minutes.
- Release pressure using the quick release method than open the lid.
- Stir well and serve.

Per Serving: Calories: 875; Total Fat: 68.3g; Saturated Fat: 31.2g; Protein: 56.6g; Carbs: 7.8g; Fiber: 2g; Sugar: 3g

Creamy Pork Chops

Serves: 6 / Preparation time: 10 minutes / Cooking time: 20 minutes

6 pastured pork chops

1 tsp onion powder

½ cup mushrooms, sliced

1 tsp chili powder

1 ½ tbsp arrowroot powder

1 cup coconut cream

2 tbsp garlic, minced

1 cup chicken broth

1 tbsp olive oil

2 tsp salt

- Add olive oil into the instant pot and set the pot on sauté mode.
- Add pork chops to the pot and sear pork chops on each side.
- Add broth and stir well. Seal pot with lid and cook on high pressure for 12 minutes.
- Release pressure using the quick release method than open the lid.
- Remove pork chops from the pot and set aside.
- Mix together arrowroot powder and coconut cream and pour into the pot and stir well.
- Set pot on sauté mode. Add onion powder, chili powder, mushrooms, garlic, and salt and cook until gravy thickens.
- Serve and enjoy.

Per Serving: Calories: 391; Total Fat: 32.1g; Saturated Fat: 16.3g; Protein: 20.2g; Carbs: 6.1g; Fiber: 1.2g; Sugar: 1.8g

Country Style Ribs

Serves: 4 / Preparation time: 10 minutes / Cooking time: 45 minutes

3 lbs pastured country style pork ribs

Dry Rub:

1 tsp onion powder

1 tsp garlic powder

3/4 cup chicken stock

1/4 tsp cayenne pepper

1 tsp cumin

1 tsp pepper

1 tsp chili powder

1 tsp salt

- In a small bowl, mix together all rub ingredients and rub over meat.
- Pour stock into the instant pot then place ribs into the pot.
- Seal pot with lid and cook on high pressure for 45 minutes.
- Allow to release pressure naturally then open the lid.
- Stir and serve.

Per Serving: Calories: 644; Total Fat: 39.5g; Saturated Fat: 13.6g; Protein: 66.8g; Carbs: 2.1g; Fiber: 0.6g; Sugar: 0.6g

Tender & Smokey Ribs

Serves: 4 / Preparation time: 10 minutes / Cooking time: 35 minutes

2 1/2 lbs pastured country-style spareribs, boneless

1 tbsp liquid smoke

14 oz chicken stock

1 tbsp sea salt

- Season spareribs with sea salt and set aside.
- Add liquid smoke and stock into the instant pot.
- Place spareribs into the pot.
- Seal pot with lid and select meat mode and set timer for 35 minutes.
- Release pressure using quick release method than open the lid.
- Serve and enjoy.

Per Serving: Calories: 782; Total Fat: 68g; Saturated Fat: 22.6g; Protein: 45.4g; Carbs: 0.3g; Fiber: 0g; Sugar: 0.3g

Chili Garlic Tip Roast

Serves: 6 / Preparation time: 10 minutes / Cooking time: 25 minutes

3 lbs pastured pork sirloin tip roast

1/2 cup apple juice

1 cup of water

1 tbsp olive oil

1/4 tsp chili powder

1/2 tsp garlic powder

1/2 tsp onion powder

1/2 tsp black pepper

1/2 tsp salt

- In a small bowl, mix together all spices.
- Rub spice mixture all over the meat.
- Add oil into the instant pot and set the pot on sauté mode.
- Add meat into the pot and sauté until brown.
- Add remaining ingredients into the pot and stir well.
- Seal pot with lid and cook on manual high pressure for 25 minutes.
- Release pressure using quick release method than open the lid.
- Serve and enjoy.

Per Serving: Calories: 234; Total Fat: 5.4g; Saturated Fat: 0.3g; Protein: 44.7g; Carbs: 2.8g; Fiber: 0.2g; Sugar: 2.1g

Mongolian Beef

Serves: 4 / Preparation time: 10 minutes / Cooking time: 25 minutes

1 1/2 lbs grass-fed flank steak, sliced

2 tbsp olive oil

1/4 cup arrowroot powder

1/2 cup carrot, grated

3/4 cup coconut aminos

1/2 tsp ginger powder

3/4 cup water

- Coat flank steak with arrowroot powder and set aside.
- Add all other ingredients into the instant pot and sauté for minutes.
- Add sliced beef and stir well.
- Cover pot with lid and cook on high pressure for 25 minutes.
- Release pressure using the quick release method than open the lid carefully.
- Stir and serve.

Per Serving: Calories: 476; Total Fat: 21.2g; Saturated Fat: 6.9g; Protein: 47.5g; Carbs: 18.5g; Fiber: 0.4g; Sugar: 0.7g

Easy Hawaiian Pork

Serves: 8 / Preparation time: 10 minutes / Cooking time: 90 minutes

5 lbs pastured pork roast, bone-in and cut into pieces

1 cup of water

5 garlic cloves, minced

1 onion, quartered

1 tbsp Hawaiian salt

Pepper

- Place meat into the instant pot.
- Add garlic, onion, pepper, and salt on top of meat. Pour water over the meat.
- Seal pot with lid and cook on high pressure for 90 minutes.
- Allow to release pressure naturally then open the lid.
- Shred the meat using a fork.
- Stir and serve.

Per Serving: Calories: 595; Total Fat: 26.8g; Saturated Fat: 9.7g; Protein: 81.1g; Carbs: 1.9g; Fiber: 0.3g; Sugar: 0.6g

Pork & Cabbage

Serves: 4 / Preparation time: 10 minutes / Cooking time: 8 minutes

1 lb pastured pork loin, boneless and cut into cubes

1/2 tsp pepper

1/2 tsp fennel seeds

1 tsp dried dill weed

1/2 small cabbage, cored and cut into wedges

1 onion, cut into wedges

2 tsp olive oil

1 tbsp white wine vinegar

1 cup chicken stock

- Add oil into the instant pot and set the pot on sauté mode.
- Add onion to the pot and sauté for 2 minutes.
- Add meat to the pot and cook for 3 minutes. Add cabbage and stir well.
- In a small bowl, mix together dill weed, pepper, and fennel seeds. Sprinkle on top of the cabbage.
- Pour vinegar and stock on top of meat mixture.
- Seal pot with lid and cook on high pressure for 5 minutes.
- Allow to release pressure naturally then open the lid.
- Serve and enjoy.

Per Serving: Calories: 333; Total Fat: 18.4g; Saturated Fat: 6.3g; Protein: 32.7g; Carbs: 8.4g; Fiber: 3g; Sugar: 4.2g

Jamaican Pork

Serves: 4 / Preparation time: 10 minutes / Cooking time: 45 minutes

2 lbs pastured pork shoulder

1 cup chicken broth

1 tbsp olive oil

2 tbsp Jamaican spice rub

- Add oil into the pot and set the pot on sauté mode.
- Add meat to the pot and cook until browned.
- Add remaining ingredients over the meat.
- Seal pot with lid and cook on high pressure for 45 minutes.
- Release pressure using quick release method than open the lid.
- Shred the meat using a fork.
- Serve and enjoy.

Per Serving: Calories: 702; Total Fat: 52.4g; Saturated Fat: 18.4g; Protein: 54g; Carbs: 0.2g; Fiber: 0g; Sugar: 0.2g

Italian Beef Roast

Serves: 6 / Preparation time: 10 minutes / Cooking time: 50 minutes

2 1/2 lbs grass-fed beef roast

2 tbsp Italian seasoning

2 tbsp olive oil

2 celery stalk, chopped

1 cup beef stock

1 cup red wine

2 garlic cloves, sliced

1 onion, sliced

- Add 1 tablespoon of olive oil into the instant pot and set the pot on sauté mode.
- Add meat into the pot and sear from all the sides.
- Transfer seared meat to a plate.
- Add remaining oil, celery, and onions to the pot and sauté for 3 minutes.
- Add seasoning and garlic and sauté for a minute.
- Return meat to the pot.
- Pour stock and red wine over the meat.
- Seal pot with lid and cook on high pressure for 40 minutes.
- Allow to release pressure naturally then open the lid.
- Serve and enjoy.

Per Serving: Calories: 277; Total Fat: 16.2g; Saturated Fat: 6.5g; Protein: 23.1g; Carbs: 3.8g; Fiber: 0.5g; Sugar: 1.6g

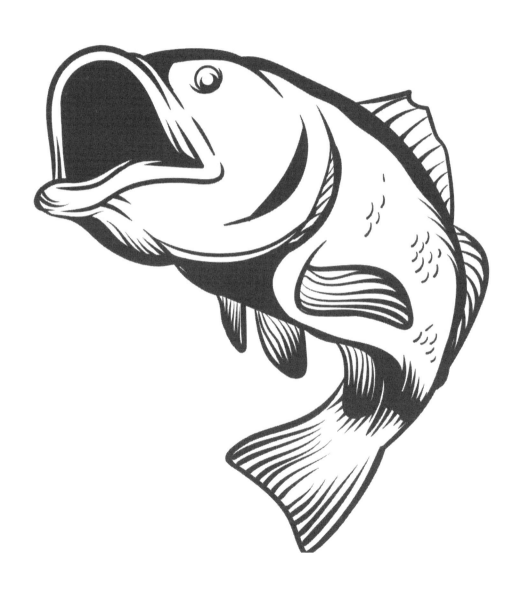

SEAFOOD RECIPES

Contents

Hearty Seafood Chowder

Serves: 6 / Preparation time: 10 minutes / Cooking time: 15 minutes

1 lb shrimp, peeled

2 lbs white fish, cut into chunks

1 lb wild salmon, cut into chunks

2 tsp dried dill

3 tsp dried parsley

3 cups chicken broth

2 cups broccoli florets

2 large sweet potato, peeled and diced

2 tsp garlic, chopped

1 large onion, chopped

1 tbsp olive oil

3 tsp salt

- Add olive oil into the instant pot and set the pot on sauté mode.
- Add garlic and onion to the pot and sauté for 5 minutes.
- Add remaining ingredients and stir well.
- Seal pot with lid and cook on manual high pressure for 10 minutes.
- Release pressure using the quick release method than open the lid.
- Stir well and serve.

Per Serving: Calories: 457; Total Fat: 13.8g; Saturated Fat: 5.4g; Protein: 50.4g; Carbs: 32.5g; Fiber: 3.4g; Sugar: 10.4g

Easy Shrimp Scampi

Serves: 2 / Preparation time: 5 minutes / Cooking time: 2 minutes

1 lb shrimp, peeled and deveined

½ lemon juice

1 cup of water

½ tsp chili powder

1 ½ tbsp garlic, minced

2 tbsp olive oil

Pepper

Salt

- Add oil into the instant pot and set the pot on sauté mode.
- Add garlic, chili powder, pepper, and salt and sauté for a minute.
- Add shrimp and water and stir well.
- Seal pot with lid and cook on high pressure for 2 minutes.
- Release pressure using the quick release method than open the lid.
- Add lemon juice and stir well.
- Serve and enjoy.

Per Serving: Calories: 404; Total Fat: 18.1g; Saturated Fat: 3.3g; Protein: 52.2g; Carbs: 6.2g; Fiber: 0.4g; Sugar: 0.4g

Curried Prawns

Serves: 2 / Preparation time: 5 minutes / Cooking time: 1 minute

1 lb king prawns, shell removed

1 tsp cumin

1 tbsp fresh coriander, chopped

1 tbsp curry paste

3 tbsp olive oil

1 tbsp garlic clove, minced

2 lime juice

Pepper

Salt

- Pour a cup of water into the instant pot then place steamer basket in the pot.
- In a large bowl, mix together lime juice, curry paste, olive oil, and garlic.
- Add prawns to the bowl and toss well.
- Add prawns into the steamer basket.
- Seal pot with lid and cook steam mode for 1 minute.
- Release pressure using the quick release method than open the lid.
- Season with pepper and salt.
- Sprinkle with cumin and chopped coriander.
- Serve and enjoy.

Per Serving: Calories: 501; Total Fat: 41.5g; Saturated Fat: 3g; Protein: 16.9g; Carbs: 14.5g; Fiber: 2.7g; Sugar: 0.8g

Nutritious Garlic Mussels

Serves: 2 / Preparation time: 10 minutes / Cooking time: 5 minutes

2 lbs mussels, scrubbed and debearded

3 tbsp fresh parsley, chopped

1 lemon juice

1 cup chicken stock

3 garlic cloves, minced

1 onion, minced

¼ cup olive oil

- Add oil into the instant pot and set the pot on sauté mode.
- Add onion and garlic to the pot and sauté for 1-2 minutes.
- Add mussels in the pot and stir well.
- Pour lemon juice and stock over the mussels.
- Seal pot with lid and cook on manual high pressure for 3 minutes.
- Release pressure using the quick release method than open the lid.
- Sprinkle with parsley and serve.

Per Serving: Calories: 647; Total Fat: 36g; Saturated Fat: 5.8g; Protein: 55.6g; Carbs: 24.6g; Fiber: 1.6g; Sugar: 3.3g

Delicious Coconut Fish Curry

Serves: 4 / Preparation time: 10 minutes / Cooking time: 5 minutes

1 lb tilapia fillets, cut into chunks

½ tsp lime juice

6 mint leaves

¼ cup cilantro, chopped

1 tsp garam masala

1 tsp cumin powder

2 tsp coriander powder

½ tsp chili powder

½ tsp turmeric

½ onion, sliced

5 curry leaves

1 tbsp ginger garlic paste

12 oz coconut milk

½ tsp mustard seeds

1 tbsp olive oil

1 tsp salt

- Add olive oil into the instant pot and set the pot on sauté mode.
- Add mustard seeds, ginger garlic paste, and curry leaves and sauté for 30 seconds.
- Add onion and sauté for 30 seconds.
- Add all spices and sauté for 30 seconds.
- Add coconut milk and stir well. Bring to simmer for a minute.
- Add tilapia, cilantro, and mint and stir well.
- Seal pot with lid and cook on manual high pressure for 2 minutes.
- Release pressure using the quick release method than open the lid.
- Add lime juice and stir well.
- Serve and enjoy.

Per Serving: Calories: 392; Total Fat: 27.7g; Saturated Fat: 19.9g; Protein: 32g; Carbs: 8g; Fiber: 3g; Sugar: 3.6g

Sea Bass Curry

Serves: 3 / Preparation time: 10 minutes / Cooking time: 3 minutes

1 lb sea bass, cut into cubes

¼ cup fresh cilantro, chopped

1 tsp ground ginger

1 tsp turmeric

2 garlic cloves, minced

2 tsp sriracha

1 tsp coconut aminos

1 tsp fish sauce

1 tbsp curry paste

1 lime juice

14.5 oz coconut milk

½ tsp white pepper

½ tsp sea salt

- In a mixing bowl, whisk together coconut milk, ginger, turmeric, garlic, sriracha, coconut aminos, fish sauce, curry paste, lime juice, pepper, and salt.
- Place sea bass into the instant pot.
- Add coconut milk. Seal pot with lid and cook on manual high pressure for 3 minutes.
- Release pressure using the quick release method than open the lid.
- Garnish with cilantro and serve.

Per Serving: Calories: 554; Total Fat: 39.6g; Saturated Fat: 30g; Protein: 39.6g; Carbs: 13.1g; Fiber: 3.5g; Sugar: 5g

Lemon Herb Salmon

Serves: 2 / Preparation time: 10 minutes / Cooking time: 3 minutes

2 salmon fillets

1 tsp dill

1 cup of water

1 lemon, sliced

½ tbsp fresh rosemary, chopped

½ tbsp parsley, chopped

½ tbsp basil, chopped

1 tsp garlic, minced

2 tbsp olive oil

2 tbsp lemon juice

Pepper

Salt

- In a small bowl, mix together olive oil, fresh herbs, garlic, and salt.
- Place salmon filets on foil and season with pepper and salt.
- Pour olive oil mixture over salmon and rub well.
- Pour lemon juice over salmon and place lemon slices on top of salmon. Cover salmon with foil.
- Pour 1 cup of water into the instant pot then place a trivet in the pot.
- Place foiled salmon on top of the trivet.
- Seal pot with lid and cook on high for 3 minutes.
- Release pressure using the quick release method than open the lid.
- Serve and enjoy.

Per Serving: Calories: 371; Total Fat: 25.3g; Saturated Fat: 3.6g; Protein: 35.1g; Carbs: 4.1g; Fiber: 1.3g; Sugar: 0.8g

Lemon Dill Tilapia

Serves: 2 / Preparation time: 10 minutes / Cooking time: 5 minutes

2 tilapia fillets

2 tbsp olive oil

4 lemon slices

2 fresh dill sprigs

½ tsp garlic powder

Pepper

Salt

- Place fish fillets on center of parchment paper.
- Season fish fillets with garlic powder, pepper, and salt.
- Place dill, lemon slices, and olive oil on top of fish fillets.
- Pour 1 cup of water into the instant pot then place a trivet in the pot.
- Cover fish fillets with parchment paper and place on top of the trivet.
- Seal pot with lid and cook on high pressure for 5 minutes.
- Release pressure using the quick release method than open the lid.
- Serve and enjoy.

Per Serving: Calories: 197; Total Fat: 15.1g; Saturated Fat: 2.5g; Protein: 16.3g; Carbs: 1.8g; Fiber: 0.5g; Sugar: 0.5g

Fish Stew

Serves: 6 / Preparation time: 10 minutes / Cooking time: 8 minutes

1 lb white fish fillets

2 tbsp olive oil

1 cup kale, chopped

1 cup cauliflower, chopped

1 cup broccoli, chopped

3 cups chicken broth

1 cup coconut cream

2 celery stalks, diced

1 carrot, sliced

1 onion, diced

Pepper

Salt

- Add olive oil into the instant pot and set the pot on sauté mode.
- Add onion to the pot and sauté for 3 minutes.
- Add all ingredients except coconut cream and stir well.
- Seal pot with lid and cook on manual high pressure for 5 minutes.
- Allow to release pressure naturally then open the lid.
- Stir in coconut cream and stir well.
- Serve and enjoy.

Per Serving: Calories: 309; Total Fat: 20.7g; Saturated Fat: 10.2g; Protein: 23.2g; Carbs: 8.6g; Fiber: 2.6g; Sugar: 3.7g

Healthy Salmon & Broccoli

Serves: 4 / Preparation time: 10 minutes / Cooking time: 4 minutes

4 salmon fillets

1 tsp garlic powder

8 oz broccoli florets

1 ½ cups water

Pepper

Salt

- Season salmon with garlic powder, pepper, and salt.
- Pour water into the instant pot then place steamer basket in the pot.
- Place salmon in the steamer basket. Add broccoli florets around the salmon.
- Seal pot with lid and cook on high pressure for 4 minutes.
- Release pressure using the quick release method than open the lid.
- Serve and enjoy.

Per Serving: Calories: 257; Total Fat: 11.2g; Saturated Fat: 1.6g; Protein: 36.2g; Carbs: 4.3g; Fiber: 1.6g; Sugar: 1.1g

Simple Dijon Fish Fillets

Serves: 4 / Preparation time: 5 minutes / Cooking time: 3 minutes

4 cod fillets

1 ½ cups water

1 ½ tbsp Dijon mustard

- Pour 1 cup of water into the instant pot then place steamer basket in the pot.
- Brush cod fillets with Dijon mustard and place in the steamer basket.
- Seal pot with lid and cook on manual high pressure for 3 minutes.
- Release pressure using the quick release method than open the lid.
- Serve and enjoy.

Per Serving: Calories: 94; Total Fat: 1.2g; Saturated Fat: 0g; Protein: 20.3g; Carbs: 0.3g; Fiber: 0.2g; Sugar: 0.1g

Creamy Lime Coconut Cod

Serves: 4 / Preparation time: 10 minutes / Cooking time: 13 minutes

1 lb cod fillets, cut into pieces

½ cup of coconut milk

¼ cup of fish sauce

1 tbsp olive oil

1 tsp garlic, minced

1 tbsp lime zest

3 tbsp almond flour

- Place fish pieces into the instant pot.
- Add remaining ingredients and stir well.
- Seal pot with lid and cook on manual mode for 10 minutes.
- Release pressure using the quick release method than open the lid.
- Set pot on sauté mode and cook for 3 minutes more.
- Serve and enjoy.

Per Serving: Calories: 228; Total Fat: 14.3g; Saturated Fat: 7g; Protein: 23g; Carbs: 3.9g; Fiber: 1.4g; Sugar: 1.9g

Lemon Prawns

Serves: 4 / Preparation time: 5 minutes / Cooking time: 3 minutes

1 lb prawns

2/3 cup chicken stock

2 tbsp fresh lemon juice

2 tbsp lemon zest

2 tbsp olive oil

2 tbsp garlic, minced

Pepper

Salt

- Add oil into the instant pot and set the pot on sauté mode.
- Add all ingredients to the pot and stir to combine.
- Seal pot with lid and cook on high pressure for 3 minutes.
- Release pressure using the quick release method than open the lid.
- Serve and enjoy.

Per Serving: Calories: 176; Total Fat: 5.6g; Saturated Fat: 1.2g; Protein: 26.3g; Carbs: 4g; Fiber: 0.3g; Sugar: 0.5g

Fish Tacos

Serves: 2 / Preparation time: 5 minutes / Cooking time: 8 minutes

2 tilapia fillets

1 1/2 tbsp ground black pepper

1 tsp olive oil

1/4 cup fresh cilantro, chopped

1 fresh lime juice

Pinch of salt

- Place fish fillets on the center of the parchment paper.
- Drizzle fish fillet with oil and lime juice. Season with pepper and salt.
- Sprinkle chopped cilantro on top of fish fillet.
- Fold parchment paper around the fish fillet and make a packet.
- Pour 1 1/2 cups of water into the instant pot then place a trivet in the pot.
- Place parchment paper packet on top of the trivet.
- Seal pot with lid and cook on high pressure for 8 minutes.
- Release pressure using quick release method than open the lid.
- Serve and enjoy.

Per Serving: Calories: 186; Total Fat: 5.2g; Saturated Fat: 1.5g; Protein: 33.2g; Carbs: 5.8g; Fiber: 2.7g; Sugar: 1.1g

Tasty Shrimp Curry

Serves: 3 / Preparation time: 5 minutes / Cooking time: 1 minute

1 lb frozen shrimp

1/2 cup water

1/8 tsp cayenne

3/4 cup onion masala

2 tbsp fresh cilantro, chopped

2 tbsp coconut milk

1/2 tsp garam masala

1/2 tsp salt

- Add all ingredients into the instant pot except coconut milk and cilantro.
- Stir well and seal pot with lid and select high pressure for 1 minute.
- Release pressure using quick release method than open the lid.
- Stir in coconut milk and garnish with cilantro.
- Serve and enjoy.

Per Serving: Calories: 184; Total Fat: 5.1g; Saturated Fat: 2.1g; Protein: 31.1g; Carbs: 2g; Fiber: 0.3g; Sugar: 0.4g

Ginger Garlic Shrimp

Serves: 4 / Preparation time: 5 minutes / Cooking time: 4 minutes

1 lb shrimp, deveined

1 tbsp ginger, minced

1/2 tsp turmeric

1 tbsp garlic, minced

7 oz unsweetened coconut milk

1/2 tsp black pepper

1 tsp garam masala

1 tsp salt

- Add all ingredients into the heat-proof bowl. Stir well and cover the bowl with foil.
- Pour 1 cup water into the instant pot then place trivet into the pot.
- Place bowl on top of the trivet.
- Seal pot with lid and cook on low pressure for 4 minutes.
- Release pressure using quick release method than open the lid.
- Serve and enjoy.

Per Serving: Calories: 258; Total Fat: 13.9g; Saturated Fat: 11.1g; Protein: 27.3g; Carbs: 6.5g; Fiber: 1.4g; Sugar: 1.7g

Quick & Easy Shrimp

Serves: 6 / Preparation time: 5 minutes / Cooking time: 1 minute

28 oz frozen shrimp, deveined

1/2 cup chicken stock

1/2 cup apple cider vinegar

- Add all ingredients into the instant pot and stir well.
- Seal pot with lid and cook on manual high pressure for 1 minute.
- Release pressure using quick release method than open the lid.
- Serve and enjoy.

Per Serving: Calories: 146; Total Fat: 2.4g; Saturated Fat: 0g; Protein: 27.1g; Carbs: 1.4g; Fiber: 0g; Sugar: 0.1g

Thai Curried Prawns

Serves: 4 / Preparation time: 10 minutes / Cooking time: 1 minute

2 lbs prawns, remove shells

3 tbsp coconut oil

1 tbsp garlic cloves, grated

2 fresh lime juice

1 tsp cumin

1 tbsp coriander

1 tbsp Thai curry paste

Pepper

Salt

- Pour 1 cup of water into the instant pot then place steamer basket in the pot.
- Add all ingredients into the large bowl and mix well.
- Add bowl mixture into the steamer basket.
- Seal pot with lid and cook on high for 1 minute.
- Release pressure using quick release method than open the lid.
- Stir well and serve.

Per Serving: Calories: 372; Total Fat: 14.2g; Saturated Fat: 10g; Protein: 52g; Carbs: 7g; Fiber: 0.2g; Sugar: 0.7g

Bok Choy Salmon

Serves: 4 / Preparation time: 10 minutes / Cooking time: 4 minutes

4 salmon fillets

2 garlic cloves, minced

2 tbsp ginger, grated

1 1/2 cups chicken stock

10 oz Bok Choy, cut into slices

1 tsp vinegar

- Add bok choy, vinegar, garlic, ginger, and stock to the instant pot and stir well.
- Place steamer rack in the instant pot and place a fish fillet in the steamer rack.
- Seal pot with lid and cook o high for 4 minutes.
- Release pressure using quick release method than open the lid.
- Transfer fish on a plate.
- Remove Bok Choy from pot and place around the salmon.
- Serve and enjoy.

Per Serving: Calories: 260; Total Fat: 11.5g; Saturated Fat: 1.7g; Protein: 36.2g; Carbs: 4.2g; Fiber: 1.1g; Sugar: 1.2g

Lemon Ginger Haddock

Serves: 2 / Preparation time: 10 minutes / Cooking time: 8 minutes

4 haddock fillets

1 cup white wine

4 green onions, chopped

1 tbsp ginger, chopped

2 tbsp olive oil

2 fresh lemon juice

Pepper

Salt

- Rub oil over the fish fillets and season with pepper and salt.
- Add all ingredients except fish fillets in the instant pot and stir well.
- Place a steamer basket in instant pot.
- Place fish in a steamer basket.
- Seal pot with lid and cook on high for 8 minutes.
- Release pressure using quick release method than open the lid.
- Serve and enjoy.

Per Serving: Calories: 584; Total Fat: 17.4g; Saturated Fat: 2.9g; Protein: 74g; Carbs: 8.3g; Fiber: 1.3g; Sugar: 2.7g

VEGETARIAN RECIPES

Contents

Citrus Brussels Sprouts

Serves: 6 / Preparation time: 10 minutes / Cooking time: 8 minutes

1 lb Brussels sprouts, trimmed halved

2 tsp orange zest

½ cup of water

½ cup of orange juice

1 tbsp olive oil

- Add oil into the pot and set the pot on sauté mode.
- Add Brussels sprouts to the pot and sauté for 3-5 minutes.
- Add orange juice and water and stir well.
- Seal pot with lid and cook on high for 3 minutes.
- Release pressure using the quick release method than open the lid.
- Garnish with orange zest and serve.

Per Serving: Calories: 63; Total Fat: 2.6g; Saturated Fat: 0.4g; Protein: 2.7g; Carbs: 9.2g; Fiber: 3g; Sugar: 3.4g

Vegan Cauliflower

Serves: 8 / Preparation time: 10 minutes / Cooking time: 1 minutes

2 lbs cauliflower, cut into florets

¼ tsp chili powder

½ tsp black pepper

½ tsp salt

- Pour 1 cup of water into the instant pot then place steamer basket in the pot.
- Add all ingredients into the large bowl and toss well.
- Transfer cauliflower mixture to the steamer basket.
- Seal pot with lid and cook on manual mode for 1 minute.
- Release pressure using the quick release method than open the lid.
- Serve and enjoy.

Per Serving: Calories: 39; Total Fat: 0.2g; Saturated Fat: 0g; Protein: 3g; Carbs: 8.2g; Fiber: 3.9g; Sugar: 3.6g

Creamy Cauliflower Mashed

Serves: 4 / Preparation time: 10 minutes / Cooking time: 4 minutes

1 cauliflower head, cut into florets

2 tbsp coconut cream

4 tbsp olive oil

3 tbsp dry ranch dressing mix

1 cup vegetable broth

- Pour broth into the instant pot then place steamer basket in the pot.
- Add cauliflower florets into the steamer basket.
- Seal pot with lid and cook on manual high pressure for 4 minutes.
- Release pressure using the quick release method than open the lid.
- Transfer cauliflower florets into the large bowl. Stir in olive oil and dressing mix and using masher mash cauliflower until getting a smooth texture.
- Stir in coconut cream.
- Serve and enjoy.

Per Serving: Calories: 167; Total Fat: 16.2g; Saturated Fat: 3.7g; Protein: 2.8g; Carbs: 4.8g; Fiber: 1.9g; Sugar: 2.3g

Kale Stir Fry

Serves: 4 / Preparation time: 10 minutes / Cooking time: 4 minutes

10 oz baby kale, wash and cut hard stems

2 tbsp water

1 onion, chopped

¼ tsp turmeric

½ tsp chili powder

2 tsp cumin seeds

1 tsp mustard seeds

2 tsp olive oil

1 tsp salt

- Add oil into the instant pot and set the pot on sauté mode.
- Add cumin seeds and mustard seeds and sauté for a minute.
- Add turmeric powder, half salt, and kale.
- Add water and stir well.
- Seal pot with lid and cook on steam mode for 1 minute.
- Release pressure using the quick release method than open the lid.
- Set pot on sauté mode.
- Add chili powder and remaining salt and sauté for 2-3 minutes.
- Serve and enjoy.

Per Serving: Calories: 78; Total Fat: 3.3g; Saturated Fat: 0.4g; Protein: 3.3g; Carbs: 11.1g; Fiber: 2.6g; Sugar: 1.3g

Kale Cauliflower Soup

Serves: 4 / Preparation time: 10 minutes / Cooking time: 15 minutes

1 large cauliflower head, chopped

2 carrots, peeled and chopped

2 cups baby kale

2 onion, sliced

½ cup of coconut milk

3 tbsp olive oil

4 cups vegetable broth

Pepper

3 garlic cloves, peeled

Salt

- Add olive oil into the instant pot and set the pot on sauté mode.
- Add onion, carrots, garlic, and salt to the pot and sauté for 5-7 minutes.
- Add cauliflower and broth and stir well.
- Seal pot with lid and cook on soup mode for 10 minutes.
- Release pressure using the quick release method than open the lid.
- Add kale and coconut milk and stir well.
- Puree the soup using an immersion blender until smooth.
- Season soup with pepper and salt.
- Serve and enjoy.

Per Serving: Calories: 299; Total Fat: 19.4g; Saturated Fat: 8.3g; Protein: 11.5g; Carbs: 24.9g; Fiber: 8.4g; Sugar: 10.6g

Stir Fry Okra

Serves: 2 / Preparation time: 10 minutes / Cooking time: 6 minutes

1 lb okra, cut into ½" pieces

3 garlic cloves, chopped

½ tsp cumin seeds

1 tbsp olive oil

1 onion, sliced

1 tsp dry mango powder

¼ tsp chili powder

1 tsp coriander powder

¼ tsp turmeric

1 tsp salt

- Add oil into the instant pot and set the pot on sauté mode.
- Add garlic and cumin seeds and sauté for 30 seconds.
- Add onion and sauté for 3 minutes.
- Add okra and spices and stir well.
- Seal pot with lid and cook on manual low pressure for 2 minutes.
- Release pressure using the quick release method than open the lid.
- Stir well and serve.

Per Serving: Calories: 183; Total Fat: 7.7g; Saturated Fat: 1.1g; Protein: 5.4g; Carbs: 24.1g; Fiber: 8.8g; Sugar: 5.8g

Healthy & Delicious Mushrooms

Serves: 4 / Preparation time: 5 minutes / Cooking time: 10 minutes

8 oz mushrooms, sliced

2 garlic cloves, minced

1 tbsp olive oil

1 cup of water

- Add mushrooms and water into the instant pot.
- Seal pot with lid and cook on manual mode for 5 minutes.
- Release pressure using the quick release method than open the lid.
- Drain mushrooms well and return in instant pot.
- Add garlic and olive oil to the mushroom and mix well.
- Set pot on sauté mode and sauté mushrooms for 5 minutes.
- Serve and enjoy.

Per Serving: Calories: 44; Total Fat: 3.7g; Saturated Fat: 0.5g; Protein: 1.9g; Carbs: 2.4g; Fiber: 0.6g; Sugar: 1g

Vegan Mushroom Soup

Serves: 4 / Preparation time: 10 minutes / Cooking time: 15 minutes

8 oz shiitake mushrooms, sliced

8 oz crimini mushrooms, sliced

2/3 cup coconut milk

3 cups vegetable broth

1 tsp dried thyme

3 garlic cloves, minced

1 carrot, peeled and chopped

1 large celery stalk, chopped

1 onion, chopped

2 tsp olive oil

½ tsp black pepper

½ tsp kosher salt

- Add olive oil into the instant pot and set the pot on sauté mode.
- Add carrots, celery, and onion to the pot and sauté for 3-4 minutes.
- Add garlic, thyme, mushrooms, and pepper and sauté for 2-3 minutes.
- Stir in vegetable broth and salt.
- Seal pot with lid and cook on high pressure for 10 minutes.
- Release pressure using the quick release method than open the lid.
- Stir in coconut milk and using immersion blender puree the soup until smooth.
- Serve and enjoy.

Per Serving: Calories: 211; Total Fat: 13.2g; Saturated Fat: 9.1g; Protein: 7.6g; Carbs: 18.7g; Fiber: 3.8g; Sugar: 7g

Mexican Mushrooms

Serves: 4 / Preparation time: 10 minutes / Cooking time: 5 minutes

1 lb white mushrooms, sliced

1 tbsp fresh lime juice

1 tbsp apple cider vinegar

¼ tsp chili powder

¼ tsp ground cumin

¼ tsp dried oregano

4 garlic cloves, chopped

3 tbsp olive oil

Salt

- Add oil into the instant pot and set the pot on sauté mode.
- Add garlic and mushrooms to the pot and cook for 2-3 minutes.
- Add remaining ingredients and stir well.
- Seal pot with lid and cook on manual high pressure for 2 minutes.
- Release pressure using the quick release method than open the lid.
- Serve and enjoy.

Per Serving: Calories: 124; Total Fat: 10.9g; Saturated Fat: 1.5g; Protein: 3.8g; Carbs: 5.9g; Fiber: 1.3g; Sugar: 2.2g

Italian Carrots

Serves: 16 / Preparation time: 10 minutes / Cooking time: 20 minutes

5 lbs baby carrots, halved

1 tsp Italian seasoning

½ cup vegetable broth

3 garlic cloves, chopped

1 onion, chopped

2 tbsp olive oil

- Add oil into the instant pot and set the pot on sauté mode.
- Add garlic and onion to the pot and sauté for 4-5 minutes.
- Add carrots and cook for 5 minutes.
- Add remaining ingredients and stir well.
- Seal pot with lid and cook on high for 10 minutes.
- Allow to release pressure naturally for 10 minutes then release using the quick release method.
- Stir well and serve.

Per Serving: Calories: 70; Total Fat: 2.1g; Saturated Fat: 0.3g; Protein: 1.2g; Carbs: 12.6g; Fiber: 4.3g; Sugar: 7.1g

Asian Mushroom Curry

Serves: 4 / Preparation time: 10 minutes / Cooking time: 27 minutes

3 cups mushrooms, sliced

¼ cup of coconut yogurt

½ cup of coconut milk

¼ tsp chili powder

¼ tsp turmeric

¼ tsp ground cumin

¼ tsp ground coriander

½ tsp garlic, minced

Salt

- Take one heatproof dish which fits into your instant pot. Add all ingredients into the dish and stir to combine.
- Pour 1 cup of water into the instant pot then place a trivet in the pot.
- Place heatproof dish on top of the trivet.
- Seal pot with lid and cook on manual high pressure for 27 minutes.
- Allow to release pressure naturally then open the lid.
- Stir well and serve.

Per Serving: Calories: 89; Total Fat: 7.6g; Saturated Fat: 6.5g; Protein: 2.7g; Carbs: 4.6g; Fiber: 1.3g; Sugar: 2.7g

Coconut Celery Soup

Serves: 4 / Preparation time: 10 minutes / Cooking time: 30 minutes

6 cups celery stalk, chopped

2 cups vegetable stock

1 onion, chopped

1/2 tsp dill

1 cup of coconut milk

1/4 tsp salt

- Add all ingredients into the instant pot and stir well.
- Seal pot with lid and cook on soup mode for 30 minutes.
- Release pressure using the quick release method than open lid carefully.
- Puree the soup using an immersion blender until smooth.
- Stir well and serve.

Per Serving: Calories: 179; Total Fat: 15.6g; Saturated Fat: 13.7g; Protein: 2.8g; Carbs: 11.5g; Fiber: 4.4g; Sugar: 6.2g

Broccoli Mash

Serves: 4 / Preparation time: 10 minutes / Cooking time: 5 minutes

1 lb broccoli, chopped

2 tbsp coconut cream

1/2 cup water

2 garlic cloves, crushed

1 tbsp olive oil

1/4 tsp pepper

1/4 tsp salt

- Add oil into the pot and set the pot on sauté mode.
- Add garlic and sauté for 30 seconds.
- Add remaining ingredients except coconut cream and stir well.
- Seal pot with lid and cook on high for 1 minute.
- Release pressure using quick release method than open the lid.
- Mash the broccoli mixture using masher until smooth.
- Stir in coconut cream. Season with pepper and salt.
- Serve and enjoy.

Per Serving: Calories: 88; Total Fat: 5.7g; Saturated Fat: 2.1g; Protein: 3.5g; Carbs: 8.5g; Fiber: 3.2g; Sugar: 2.2g

Creamy Cauliflower Soup

Serves: 6 / Preparation time: 10 minutes / Cooking time: 10 minutes

1 lb cauliflower florets

3 garlic cloves, minced

1 onion, sliced

3 cups vegetable stock

1 cup of coconut milk

1 tbsp olive oil

2 tsp salt

- Add oil into the instant pot and set the pot on sauté mode.
- Add onion into the pot and sauté until softened.
- Add cauliflower and garlic and sauté for 5 minutes.
- Pour coconut milk and stock into the instant pot and stir well.
- Seal pot with lid and cook on soup mode for 5 minutes.
- Allow to release pressure naturally then open the lid.
- Puree the soup using an immersion blender until smooth.
- Serve and enjoy.

Per Serving: Calories: 142; Total Fat: 12.3g; Saturated Fat: 9.1g; Protein: 2.7g; Carbs: 8.8g; Fiber: 3.2g; Sugar: 4.3g

Healthy Carrot Broccoli Soup

Serves: 4 / Preparation time: 10 minutes / Cooking time: 30 minutes

2 small carrots, diced

2 celery stalk, sliced

2 cups broccoli florets, chopped

1 onion, diced

1 cup coconut cream

32 oz vegetable broth

2 tbsp olive oil

1/2 tsp pepper

1/2 tsp salt

- Add olive oil into the instant pot and set the pot on sauté mode.
- Add onion, carrots, and celery into the pot and sauté until tender.
- Add remaining ingredients except for coconut cream into the pot and stir well.
- Seal pot with lid and cook on soup mode for 30 minutes.
- Allow to release pressure naturally then open the lid.
- Add coconut cream and stir well.
- Serve and enjoy.

Per Serving: Calories: 273; Total Fat: 22.8g; Saturated Fat: 14g; Protein: 7.8g; Carbs: 12.7g; Fiber: 3.9g; Sugar: 5.9g

Lemon Coconut Cabbage

Serves: 4 / Preparation time: 10 minutes / Cooking time: 19 minutes

1 medium cabbage, shredded

1/3 cup water

1/2 cup desiccated coconut

2 tbsp lemon juice

1/2 red chili, sliced

2 garlic cloves, diced

1 carrot, sliced

1 tbsp turmeric powder

1 tbsp curry powder

1 tbsp mustard seeds

1 onion, sliced

1 tbsp olive oil

1 1/2 tsp salt

- Add oil into the instant pot and set the pot on sauté mode.
- Add onion and salt and sauté for 2-3 minutes.
- Add spices, chili, and garlic and stir for 30 seconds.
- Add carrots, cabbage, coconut, and lime juice. Stir well.
- Pour water into the pot and stir well.
- Seal pot with lid and cook on high for 5 minutes.
- Allow to release pressure naturally for 10 minutes then release using the quick release method.
- Stir and serve.

Per Serving: Calories: 162; Total Fat: 8.5g; Saturated Fat: 1.3g; Protein: 4.5g; Carbs: 20.9g; Fiber: 8g; Sugar: 9.6g

Easy Cauliflower Rice

Serves: 4 / Preparation time: 10 minutes / Cooking time: 3 minutes

1 medium cauliflower head, cut into florets

2 tbsp olive oil

1/4 tsp chili powder

1/4 tsp turmeric

1/4 tsp cumin

1/2 tsp dried parsley

1/4 tsp salt

- Pour 1 cup of water into the instant pot then place steamer basket in the pot.
- Add cauliflower florets into the steamer basket.
- Seal pot with lid and cook on manual high pressure for 1 minute.
- Release pressure using quick release method than open the lid.
- Remove cauliflower from pot and place on a dish.
- Remove water from the instant pot.
- Add olive oil into the pot and set the pot on sauté mode.
- Add cooked cauliflower florets to the instant pot and stir well.
- Break the cauliflower using potato masher into the small pieces.
- Add remaining ingredients and stir well and cook on sauté mode for 1-2 minutes.
- Serve and enjoy.

Per Serving: Calories: 97; Total Fat: 7.2g; Saturated Fat: 1g; Protein: 2.9g; Carbs: 7.9g; Fiber: 3.7g; Sugar: 3.5g

Simple Braised Cabbage

Serves: 2 / Preparation time: 10 minutes / Cooking time: 8 minutes

1 1/2 lbs cabbage, sliced into strips

1 tbsp olive oil

1 onion, sliced

1/2 cup vegetable stock

- Add oil into the pot and set the pot on sauté mode.
- Add onion and sauté for 5 minutes.
- Add cabbage and stock and stir well.
- Seal pot with lid and cook on high for 3 minutes.
- Release pressure using quick release method than open the lid.
- Stir well and serve.

Per Serving: Calories: 170; Total Fat: 7.9g; Saturated Fat: 1.6g; Protein: 5g; Carbs: 25.4g; Fiber: 9.7g; Sugar: 13.7g

Mint Baby Carrots

Serves: 4 / Preparation time: 5 minutes / Cooking time: 3 minutes

16 oz baby carrots

1 tbsp olive oil

1 tbsp fresh mint leaves, chopped

1 cup of water

Sea salt

- Add carrots and water into the instant pot.
- Seal pot with lid and cook on high for 2 minutes.
- Release pressure using quick release method than open the lid.
- Drain carrots well. Clean the instant pot.
- Add olive oil and mint into the pot and sauté for 30 seconds.
- Return carrots to the pot and season with salt.
- Stir well and serve.

Per Serving: Calories: 70; Total Fat: 3.7g; Saturated Fat: 0.5g; Protein: 0.8g; Carbs: 9.5g; Fiber: 3.4g; Sugar: 5.4g

Healthy Spinach Soup

Serves: 2 / Preparation time: 10 minutes / Cooking time: 10 minutes

3 cups spinach, chopped

1 tsp garlic powder

2 tbsp olive oil

½ cup coconut cream

3 cups chicken broth

1 cup cauliflower, chopped

½ tsp black pepper

¼ tsp sea salt

- Add olive oil into the instant pot and set the pot on sauté mode.
- Add cauliflower, spinach, garlic powder, pepper, and salt to the pot and stir well.
- Add broth and stir well.
- Seal pot with lid and cook on manual high pressure for 10 minutes.
- Allow to release pressure naturally for 10 minutes then release using the quick release method.
- Puree the soup using an immersion blender until smooth.
- Stir in coconut cream. Season with pepper and salt.
- Serve and enjoy.

Per Serving: Calories: 344; Total Fat: 30.6g; Saturated Fat: 15.3g; Protein: 11.2g; Carbs: 10.3g; Fiber: 3.8g; Sugar: 4.8g

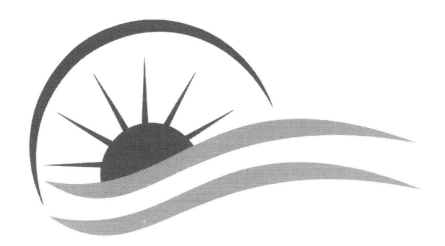

BREAKFAST RECIPES

Contents

Hearty Mushroom Frittata

Serves: 4 / Preparation time: 10 minutes / Cooking time: 30 minutes

4 pastured large eggs

1 tsp dried thyme

½ cup coconut cream

8 oz mushrooms, sliced

1 tbsp olive oil

1 tsp salt

- Spray spring-form pan with cooking spray and set aside.
- Add olive oil into the instant pot and set the pot on sauté mode.
- Add mushrooms to the pot and sauté for 5 minutes. Transfer sautéed mushroom to the prepared pan.
- In a large bowl, whisk eggs and coconut cream until light. Add thyme and salt and mix well.
- Pour egg mixture into the pan over sautéed mushrooms. Cover pan with foil.
- Pour 1 ½ cups of water into the instant pot then place a trivet in the pot.
- Place spring-form pan on top of the trivet.
- Seal pot with lid and cook on manual high pressure for 25 minutes.
- Allow to release pressure naturally for 10 minutes then release using the quick release method.
- Carefully remove the pan from the pot.
- Slice and serve.

Per Serving: Calories: 183; Total Fat: 15.8g; Saturated Fat: 8.4g; Protein: 8.8g; Carbs: 4.1g; Fiber: 1.3g; Sugar: 2.4g

Scrambled Eggs

Serves: 4 / Preparation time: 10 minutes / Cooking time: 6 minutes

4 pastured eggs

½ tsp allspice

2 tsp cinnamon

2 tbsp olive oil

¼ tsp black pepper

1/8 tsp salt

- Add olive oil into the instant pot and set the pot on sauté mode.
- In a mixing bowl, add eggs and beat until light.
- Add allspice, cinnamon, pepper, and salt.
- Add egg mixture to the pot and cook for 2 minutes. Scramble the eggs using a spatula.
- Seal pot with lid and cook on manual high pressure for 4 minutes.
- Release pressure using the quick release method than open the lid.
- Serve and enjoy.

Per Serving: Calories: 134; Total Fat: 11.5g; Saturated Fat: 2.5g; Protein: 6.1g; Carbs: 2.2g; Fiber: 0.7g; Sugar: 0g

Broccoli Frittata

Serves: 4 / Preparation time: 10 minutes / Cooking time: 20 minutes

6 pastured eggs

1/3 cup coconut milk

½ cup broccoli florets, chopped

¼ cup fresh dill, chopped

1/3 cup goat cheese, crumbled

Pepper

Salt

- In a bowl, beat eggs, with broccoli, coconut milk, dill, and goat cheese.
- Transfer egg mixture into a greased 7-inch spring-form pan. Cover pan with foil.
- Pour 2 cups of water into the instant pot then place a trivet in the pot.
- Place spring-form pan on top of the trivet.
- Seal pot with lid and cook on manual high pressure for 20 minutes.
- Allow to release pressure naturally for 10 minutes then release using the quick release method.
- Serve and enjoy.

Per Serving: Calories: 223; Total Fat: 16.3g; Saturated Fat: 9.5g; Protein: 14.4g; Carbs: 5.8g; Fiber: 1.2g; Sugar: 0.9g

Spinach Frittata

Serves: 6 / Preparation time: 10 minutes / Cooking time: 10 minutes

7 pastured large eggs

1 cup of water

1 ½ cups baby spinach, chopped

½ tsp nutmeg, grated

2 tbsp coconut cream

Pepper

Salt

- In a bowl, beat eggs with nutmeg, coconut cream, pepper, and salt until smooth.
- Add spinach and stir well.
- Spray 7-inch spring-form pan with cooking spray.
- Pour egg mixture into the prepared pan.
- Pour 1 cup of water into the instant pot then place a trivet in the pot.
- Place pan on top of the trivet.
- Seal pot with lid and cook on high pressure for 10 minutes.
- Release pressure using the quick release method than open the lid.
- Serve and enjoy.

Per Serving: Calories: 96; Total Fat: 6.5g; Saturated Fat: 2.8g; Protein:7.4g; Carbs: 1.8g; Fiber: 0.3g; Sugar: 0.3g

Spinach Mushroom Frittata

Serves: 6 / Preparation time: 10 minutes / Cooking time: 30 minutes

8 pastured eggs

2 tbsp coconut milk

1 tbsp fresh lemon juice

¼ cup goat cheese, crumbled

6 oz baby spinach, rinsed

2 garlic cloves, minced

½ onion, chopped

8 oz mushrooms, sliced

2 tbsp olive oil

¼ tsp black pepper

Salt

- Heat olive oil in a pan over medium-high heat.
- Add onion and mushrooms to the pan and sauté for 3 minutes.
- Add garlic, lemon juice, pepper, and salt and sauté for 30 seconds.
- In a large bowl, beat eggs.
- Add cheese, milk, and mushrooms mixture to the eggs and stir well.
- Add spinach to the egg mixture and stir well.
- Pour egg mixture into the 7-inch greased pan.
- Pour 2 cups of water into the instant pot then place a trivet in the pot.
- Place pan on top of the trivet.
- Seal pot with lid and cook on manual high pressure for 25 minutes.
- Allow to release pressure naturally for 10 minutes then release using the quick release method.
- Serve and enjoy.

Per Serving: Calories: 285; Total Fat: 21.4g; Saturated Fat: 9.7g; Protein: 18.3g; Carbs: 6.5g; Fiber: 1.4g; Sugar: 1.4g

Brussels sprouts with Pine Nut

Serves: 4 / Preparation time: 5 minutes / Cooking time: 3 minutes

1 lb Brussels sprouts

1 cup of water

1/2 tbsp olive oil

1/4 cup pine nuts

Pepper

Salt

- Pour water into the instant pot.
- Add Brussels sprouts in steamer basket and place basket in the pot.
- Seal pot with lid and cook on manual high pressure for 3 minutes.
- Release pressure using the quick release method. Open the lid carefully.
- Season with pepper and salt. Drizzle with olive oil.
- Sprinkle pine nuts and serve.

Per Serving: Calories: 121; Total Fat: 8g; Saturated Fat: 0.8g; Protein: 5g; Carbs: 11.4g; Fiber: 4.6g; Sugar: 2.8g

Healthy Carrot with Raisins

Serves: 4 / Preparation time: 5 minutes / Cooking time: 3 minutes

1 lb carrots, peeled and sliced

1 tbsp coconut oil

1 cup of water

3 tbsp raisins

1/2 tsp pepper

- Add water, carrots, and raisins into the instant pot.
- Seal pot with lid and cook on high for 3 minutes.
- Release pressure using the quick release method than open lid carefully.
- Drain carrot well and transfer in a bowl.
- Add coconut oil in a bowl and toss well until oil is melted.
- Season with black pepper.
- Serve and enjoy.

Per Serving: Calories: 97; Total Fat: 3.4g; Saturated Fat: 2.9g; Protein: 1.2g; Carbs: 16.7g; Fiber: 3.1g; Sugar: 9.6g

Delicious Korean Egg

Serves: 1 / Preparation time: 5 minutes / Cooking time: 5 minutes

1 egg

1/8 tsp sesame seeds

1 tsp scallions, chopped

1/3 cup water

1/8 tsp garlic powder

Pepper

Salt

- In a small bowl, whisk together egg and water.
- Strain egg mixture over a fine strainer into a heat safe bowl.
- Add remaining ingredients and mix well. Set aside.
- Pour 1 cup water into the instant pot and then place trivet into the pot.
- Place egg bowl on a trivet. Seal pot with lid and cook on high pressure for 5 minutes.
- Release pressure using the quick release method than open the lid carefully.
- Serve and enjoy.

Per Serving: Calories: 67; Total Fat: 4.6g; Saturated Fat: 1.4g; Protein: 5.7g; Carbs: 0.9g; Fiber: 0.2g; Sugar: 0.5g

Healthy Carrot Muffins

Serves: 8 / Preparation time: 10 minutes / Cooking time: 20 minutes

3 eggs

1 1/2 cups water

1/2 cup coconut cream

1 tsp apple pie spice

1/4 cup coconut oil, melted

1 cup almond flour

1/2 cup pecans, chopped

1 cup shredded carrot

1/3 cup Truvia

1 tsp baking powder

- Pour water into the instant pot then place a trivet in the pot.
- Add all ingredients except pecans and carrots into the large bowl and using electric mixer blend until fluffy.
- Add carrots and pecans and fold well.
- Pour batter into the silicone muffin cups and place on top of the trivet.
- Seal pot with lid and cook on high for 20 minutes.
- Release pressure using quick release method than open the lid.
- Serve and enjoy.

Per Serving: Calories: 256; Total Fat: 24.6g; Saturated Fat: 10.6g; Protein: 6.3g; Carbs: 9.9g; Fiber: 3g; Sugar: 5.2g

Steamed Broccoli

Serves: 2 / Preparation time: 5 minutes / Cooking time: 1 minutes

3 cups broccoli head, cut into florets

2 garlic cloves, peeled and crushed

1 cup vegetable stock

Pepper

Salt

- Pour stock into the instant pot.
- Add all ingredients into the instant pot steamer basket and place in the pot.
- Seal pot with lid and cook on low for 1 minute.
- Release pressure using quick release method than open the lid.
- Serve and enjoy.

Per Serving: Calories: 56; Total Fat: 1.5g; Saturated Fat: 1g; Protein: 4g; Carbs: 11.1g; Fiber: 3.6g; Sugar: 3.4g

Creamy Cauliflower Mash

Serves: 8 / Preparation time: 10 minutes / Cooking time: 3 minutes

1 cauliflower head, chopped

2 tbsp coconut yogurt

1/2 cup vegetable broth

2 tbsp fresh chives, chopped

2 tsp coconut oil, melted

Pepper

Salt

- Pour broth into the instant pot and place steamer basket in the pot.
- Add cauliflower into the steamer basket.
- Seal pot with lid and cook on high for 3 minutes.
- Release pressure using quick release method than open the lid.
- Transfer cauliflower into the food processor along with coconut yogurt, pepper and salt and process until smooth.
- Drizzle with melted coconut oil and garnish with chives.
- Serve and enjoy.

Per Serving: Calories: 22; Total Fat: 1.3g; Saturated Fat: 1g; Protein: 1g; Carbs: 2.1g; Fiber: 0.9g; Sugar: 1.1g

Spicy Cinnamon Carrots

Serves: 4 / Preparation time: 10 minutes / Cooking time: 1 minutes

1 lb carrots, halved and quartered

1/8 tsp cinnamon

1/4 tsp chili powder

3 tsp ground mustard

2 tbsp coconut oil

1 tbsp swerve

1/2 tsp black pepper

1 tsp ground cumin

Salt

- Pour 1 cup of water into the instant pot and place steamer basket in the pot.
- Add carrots in the steamer basket.
- Seal pot with lid and cook on high for 1 minute.
- Release pressure using quick release method than open the lid.
- Transfer carrots to the bowl.
- Remove water from the pot.
- Add coconut oil into the instant pot and set the pot on sauté mode.
- Add remaining ingredients and stir well.
- Add carrots and stir for 1 minute.
- Turn off the instant pot.
- Sprinkle cinnamon on top of carrots and serve.

Per Serving: Calories: 120; Total Fat: 7.7g; Saturated Fat: 5.9g; Protein: 1.7g; Carbs: 16.3g; Fiber: 3.4g; Sugar: 9.5g

Sweet Cinnamon Carrots

Serves: 8 / Preparation time: 10 minutes / Cooking time: 4 minutes

2 lbs baby carrots

1/2 cup water

1/2 tsp ground cinnamon

2 tbsp swerve

1/3 cup coconut oil

Salt

- Add all ingredients into the instant pot and stir to combine.
- Seal pot with lid and cook on high for 4 minutes.
- Allow to release pressure naturally then open the lid.
- Serve and enjoy.

Per Serving: Calories: 118; Total Fat: 9.2g; Saturated Fat: 7.9g; Protein: 0.7g; Carbs: 13.2g; Fiber: 3.4g; Sugar: 9.2g

Lemon Muffins

Serves: 4 / Preparation time: 10 minutes / Cooking time: 15 minutes

1 egg

¼ cup of coconut milk

1 tsp coconut oil, melted

1 tbsp poppy seeds

1 tbsp swerve

1 tbsp lemon juice

¼ tsp lemon zest

1 cup coconut flour

Pinch of salt

- Pour 1 ½ cups of water into the instant pot then place a trivet in the pot.
- In a bowl, combine together all dry ingredients.
- In another bowl whisk together all wet ingredients.
- Slowly add dry mixture into the wet mixture and mix until well combined.
- Pour batter into four silicone muffin cups.
- Place muffin cups on top of the trivet.
- Seal pot with lid and cook on high for 15 minutes.
- Release pressure using the quick release method than open the lid.
- Serve and enjoy.

Per Serving: Calories: 88; Total Fat: 7.3g; Saturated Fat: 5.1g; Protein: 2.7g; Carbs: 7.3g; Fiber: 1.8g; Sugar: 5g

Coconut Porridge

Serves: 6 / Preparation time: 10 minutes / Cooking time: 1 minutes

1 cup shredded coconut

15 drops monk fruit liquid

25 drops liquid stevia

¼ tsp nutmeg

½ tsp cinnamon

1 tsp vanilla

¼ cup psyllium husks

¼ cup coconut flour

2 2/3 cups water

2 cups of coconut milk

- Add water, coconut milk, and shredded coconut into the instant pot and stir well.
- Seal pot with lid and cook on high pressure for 1 minute.
- Allow to release pressure naturally for 10 minutes then release using the quick release method.
- Add remaining ingredients and stir well.
- Serve and enjoy.

Per Serving: Calories: 293; Total Fat: 23.6g; Saturated Fat: 21g; Protein: 2.4g; Carbs: 29.6g; Fiber: 22g; Sugar: 3.7g

Spinach Cheese Omelet

Serves: 1 / Preparation time: 10 minutes / Cooking time: 16 minutes

3 pastured eggs, beaten

1 ½ cups water

¼ tsp garlic salt

1 oz goat cheese

2 cups spinach

1 spring onion, chopped

¼ cup onion, sliced

2 tbsp coconut oil, melted

Pepper

Salt

- Add coconut oil into the instant pot and set the pot on sauté mode.
- Add onion to the pot and sauté for 3 minutes.
- Stir in spinach and spices and cook for a minute.
- Transfer mixture to a greased baking dish.
- Add egg mixture over spinach mixture. Stir in goat cheese.
- Pour water into the instant pot then place a trivet in the pot.
- Place baking dish on top of the trivet.
- Seal pot with lid and cook on high for 12 minutes.
- Release pressure using the quick release method than open the lid.
- Serve and enjoy.

Per Serving: Calories: 605; Total Fat: 51.1g; Saturated Fat: 35g; Protein: 29.2g; Carbs: 10.2g; Fiber: 2.4g; Sugar: 2.6g

Simple Steamed Cauliflower

Serves: 2 / Preparation time: 5 minutes / Cooking time: 1 minutes

1 cauliflower head, cut into florets

1 cup vegetable stock

½ tsp onion powder

¼ tsp garlic powder

Pepper

Salt

- Pour water into the instant pot then place steamer basket in the pot.
- Add cauliflower florets into the steamer basket.
- Seal pot with lid and cook on high pressure for 1 minute.
- Allow to release pressure naturally for 10 minutes then release using the quick release method than open the lid.
- Transfer cauliflower florets to the large bowl. Season with onion powder, garlic powder, pepper, and salt.
- Serve and enjoy.

Per Serving: Calories: 42; Total Fat: 1.1g; Saturated Fat: 1g; Protein: 2.8g; Carbs: 8.8g; Fiber: 3.4g; Sugar: 4.5g

Perfect Sweet Potato Mash

Serves: 6 / Preparation time: 5 minutes / Cooking time: 10 minutes

3 lbs sweet potatoes, peeled and cut into chunks

1 cup vegetable stock

½ tsp black pepper

½ tsp salt

- Add all ingredients into the instant pot and stir well.
- Seal pot with lid and cook on manual high pressure for 10 minutes.
- Allow to release pressure naturally for 5 minutes then release using the quick release method than open the lid.
- Using potato masher mash sweet potato until smooth.
- Serve and enjoy.

Per Serving: Calories: 270; Total Fat: 0.7g; Saturated Fat: 0.4g; Protein: 3.5g; Carbs: 63.7g; Fiber: 9.4g; Sugar: 1.5g

Easy & Hearty Sauerkraut

Serves: 8 / Preparation time: 10 minutes / Cooking time: 14 minutes

28 oz shredded sauerkraut

½ tsp black pepper

¾ tsp caraway seeds

½ cup vegetable broth

1 onion, chopped

1 tbsp olive oil

- Add olive oil into the instant pot and set the pot on sauté mode.
- Add onion to the pot and sauté for 4 minutes.
- Add broth and stir well.
- Add remaining ingredients and stir until mix.
- Seal pot with lid and cook on manual high pressure for 10 minutes.
- Allow to release pressure naturally for 10 minutes then release using the quick release method.
- Stir well and serve.

Per Serving: Calories: 43; Total Fat: 2g; Saturated Fat: 0.3g; Protein: 1.4g; Carbs: 5.8g; Fiber: 3.3g; Sugar: 2.4g

Mushroom Omelet

Serves: 5 / Preparation time: 5 minutes / Cooking time: 10 minutes

5 pastured eggs

2 tbsp coconut oil

½ tbsp goat cheese, crumbled

1 onion, chopped

2 tbsp fresh chives, chopped

1 ½ cups mushrooms, sliced

½ cup of coconut milk

Pepper

Salt

- Add oil into the instant pot and set the pot on sauté mode.
- In a bowl, whisk eggs until light. Add remaining ingredients and mix well.
- Transfer egg mixture to the instant pot and cook for 2 minutes.
- Seal pot with lid and cook on manual high pressure for 8 minutes.
- Release pressure using the quick release method than open the lid.
- Serve and enjoy.

Per Serving: Calories: 190; Total Fat: 16.1g; Saturated Fat: 11.5g; Protein: 7.8g; Carbs: 5.2g; Fiber: 1.3g; Sugar: 2.1g

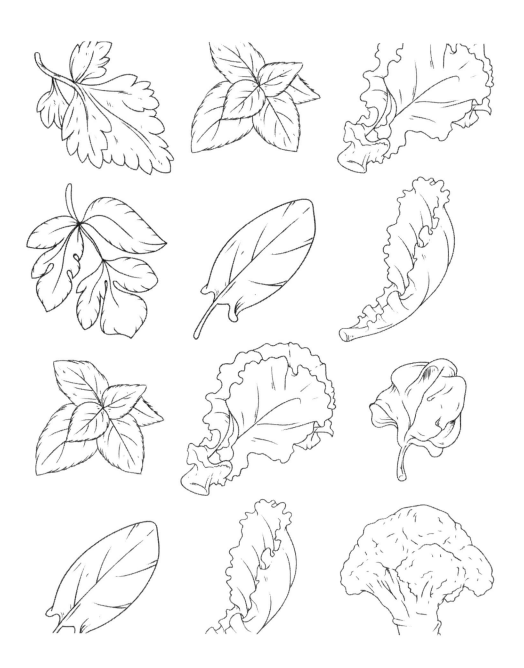

THE "DIRTY DOZEN" AND "CLEAN 15"

Every year, the Environmental Working Group releases a list of the produce with the most pesticide residue (Dirty Dozen) and a list of the ones with the least **chance of having residue (Clean 15). It's based on analysis from the U.S.** Department of Agriculture Pesticide Data Program report.

The Environmental Working Group found that 70% of the 48 types of produce tested had residues of at least one type of pesticide. In total there were 178 different pesticides and pesticide breakdown products. This residue can stay on veggies and fruit even after they are washed and peeled. All pesticides are toxic to humans and consuming them can cause damage to the nervous system, reproductive system, cancer, a weakened immune system, and more. Women who are pregnant can expose their unborn children to toxins through their diet, and continued exposure to pesticides can affect their development.

This info can help you choose the best fruits and veggies, as well as which ones you should always try to buy organic.

The Dirty Dozen

- Strawberries
- Spinach
- Nectarines
- Apples
- Peaches
- Celery
- Grapes
- Pears
- Cherries
- Tomatoes
- Sweet bell peppers
- Potatoes

The Clean 15

- Sweet corn
- Avocados
- Pineapples
- Cabbage
- Onions
- Frozen sweet peas
- Papayas
- Asparagus
- Mangoes
- Eggplant
- Honeydew
- Kiwi
- Cantaloupe
- Cauliflower
- Grapefruit

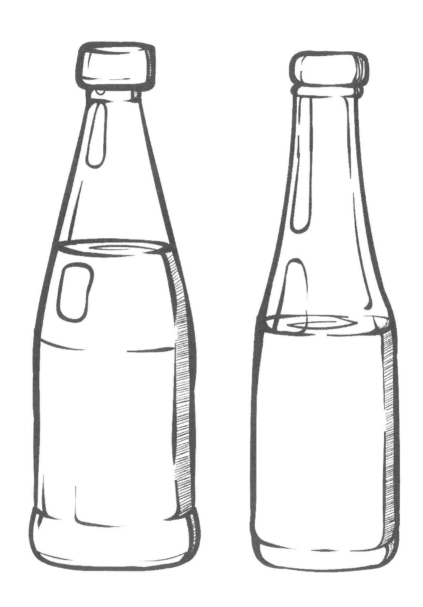

MEASUREMENT CONVERSION TABLES

Volume Equivalents (Dry)

US Standard	Metric (Approx.)
¼ teaspoon	1 ml
½ teaspoon	2 ml
1 teaspoon	5 ml
1 tablespoon	15 ml
¼ cup	59 ml
½ cup	118 ml
1 cup	235 ml

Weight Equivalents

US Standard	Metric (Approx.)
½ ounce	15 g
1 ounce	30 g
2 ounces	60 g
4 ounces	115 g
8 ounces	225 g
12 ounces	340 g
16 oz or 1 lb	455 g

Volume Equivalents (Liquid)

US Standard	US Standard (ounces)	Metric (Approx.)
2 tablespoons	1 fl oz	30 ml
¼ cup	2 fl oz	60 ml
½ cup	4 fl oz	120 ml
1 cup	8 fl oz	240 ml
1 ½ cups	12 fl oz	355 ml
2 cups or 1 pint	16 fl oz	475 ml
4 cups or 1 quart	32 fl oz	1 L
1 gallon	128 fl oz	4 L

Oven Temperatures

Fahrenheit (F)	Celsius (C) (Approx)
250°F	120°C
300°F	150°C
325°F	165°C
350°F	180°C
375°F	190°C
400°F	200°C
425°F	220°C
450°F	230°C

INDEX

Manufactured by Amazon.ca
Bolton, ON